THE **SECRETS** OF
UNDERGROUND
MEDICINE

DR. RICHARD GERHAUSER, M.D.

Natural Health Response

CONTENTS

CANCER-CONQUERING SECRETS FROM THE MEDICAL UNDERGROUND

MAKE PAIN VANISH WITH THESE AMAZING TRICKS

HEAL YOUR HEART WITH THESE SIMPLE (AND SAFE) TRICKS

HOW TO BEAT DIABETES WITHOUT A PRESCRIPTION

ALL-NATURAL SOLUTIONS FOR PERFECT SLEEP

LIVE LONGER (AND LOOK YOUNGER) WITH THESE UNDERGROUND BREAKTHROUGHS

10 MORE LIFE-CHANGING BONUS TIPS!

CHAPTER ONE

SUPER BRAIN SECRETS FOR SENIORS

REVERSE MEMORY LOSS WITH THIS "BRAIN SURGE PROTOCOL"

Those "senior moments" can be some of the most frightening parts of aging. You know what I'm talking about.

Maybe you've walked into a room and completely forgotten why you were there… or perhaps you've misplaced your car keys or wallet more times than you can count.

For years you've probably been told that it's a normal part of aging, and that there's nothing you can do about it anyway.

But there's a lot more to this story that you haven't been told.

You see, these senior moments can actually be symptoms of a larger problem called "mild cognitive impairment," or MCI. And in 34 percent of cases, MCI progresses to full-blown Alzheimer's.

That's not a gamble I'm willing to take with your health… and I bet you're not willing to take it either.

That's why I'm going to introduce you to my 5-step "Brain Surge Protocol" that can protect your precious memories and actually reverse MCI before it's too late.

But first I need you to set aside everything… and I mean everything… that the mainstream medical establishment has ever taught us about memory loss.

The TRUTH About Brain Drain

As long as I've been practicing medicine, Big Pharma has been trying to invent some magical memory pill.

They've failed every single time, and for a very good reason. They simply don't understand the problem.

You see, there's a very important cellular disorder that may be causing your memory loss. It usually goes undiagnosed and even many mainstream doctors don't understand it.

And that's a real shame, because this condition is actually completely reversible.

Let me explain. I'm sure at one point or another, you or your kids owned some battery-powered toys.

And you remember what would happen when the batteries started to fail, right? The toy would still work, but it was slow… or even lethargic.

Maybe your brain feels that way sometimes, too. And that makes complete sense, because something very similar is happening.

Thanks to the research efforts of Dr. Doug Wallace and his colleagues, we know more than ever about something called "cellular energetics," or how our cells use energy.

Dr. Wallace estimates that 85 percent of degenerative diseases, including MCI and dementia, are due to problems with energy production in the mitochondria, which are like the power plants of our cells.

In other words, our brains are literally starving for energy!

The typical neuron cell in our brains will contain over 3,000 mitochondria. And all of these mitochondria have 13 key genes that are responsible for transferring electricity, the source of energy that keeps us alive and keeps our brains functioning properly.

So, when your mitochondria are healthy, they are literally humming with energy and your brain feels sharp as a tack.

When your mitochondria stop working properly, you develop what's known as mitochondrial heteroplasmy. That's when your mitochondrial DNA get damaged, and heteroplasmy rates increase as we age.

When you're suffering from heteroplasmy, your mito-chondria have poor energy production and leave you suscep-tible to degenerative diseases like MCI or even dementia. Your brain becomes like that toy with the failing batteries.

The good news is that there's plenty you can do… starting today… to improve mitochondrial function and give your brain all the energy it needs.

That's why I developed this 5-step Brain Surge Protocol to help reverse cognitive impairment and preserve the memories you've spent a lifetime building.

The Brain Surge Protocol

The best part of my Brain Surge Protocol is that it doesn't require any dangerous prescription drugs.

And, because it mostly involves simple lifestyle changes, it's easy to follow, even on a limited budget.

Just follow these steps, and I guarantee you're going to feel your memory improve in a matter of weeks.

Step #1: Protect Your Brain's Inner Clock

You may have heard before that poor sleep is actually a major risk factor for cognitive decline. But, really, the problem goes much deeper than that to something known as our circadian rhythm.

Your circadian rhythm is like your body's own internal

clock, which follows the day/night cycle and tells us when to be awake and when to sleep.

It's controlled by proteins and peptides that direct the millions of chemical reactions in our cells and in our mitochondria.

Research proves that a healthy circadian rhythm is critical to keeping your mitochondria working correctly and heading off memory loss.

But there's one BIG problem. Our constant exposure to artificial light, especially at night, actually fouls up our circadian rhythm and can damage our mitochondria (I'll explain more later in this chapter).

You need your body's internal clock to follow the Earth's day/night cycle as closely as possible. This means getting your eyes and skin exposed to natural sunlight daily.

This also means mitigating the effects of man-made light, particularly blue light from electronic devices and energy efficient light bulbs.

Keep your bedroom completely dark at night. Ban the TV and computer from the bedroom, and download a blue light filter for your phone (you'll find them at just about any app store).

It's amazing how many patients I've seen who experience memory improvements just by getting more sunlight and less artificial light. It's like the mitochondria in their brain cells spring back to life!

Step #2: Load Up On This Key Brain Nutrient

One of the most important nutrients needed for healthy brain mitochondria is docosahexaenoic acid, or DHA. It's one of the omega-3 fish oils.

DHA has its highest concentration in tissues of the brain and the retinas of our eyes. And it has the unique ability to interact with light to produce an electric current that sends a signal in our nervous system and other tissues.

Simply put, it helps produce energy that the starving mitochondria in our brain cells crave.

Now, there are some doctors out there who will tell you that taking fish oil supplements is as good as eating fish. Well, I guess I'm not one of them.

There are plenty of brain-healthy nutrients in fish other than DHA. For example, crab, lobster and shrimp shells contain astaxanthin, which is an important brain protecting food.

Seafood also is a good source of iodine, vitamin A and selenium which are important for optimal brain functioning.

Step #3: Help Your Body Build New Mitochondria

Part of staving off memory loss... and keeping your brain cells' mitochondria supplied with energy... is a process called mitophagy.

That's when your body produces new, healthy mitochondria.

And there's a simple way to do it — just make sure you're getting exercise every day. Research shows that exercise actually stimulates mitophagy, which keeps your brain's mitochondria in tip-top shape.

This is really important, because as some people begin to suffer from memory loss, they stop exercising and basically become shut-ins.

Now they're missing out on some of the key elements (like more sunlight, less artificial light, and more exercise) that can actually help their brains improve.

If you want to beat memory loss, you absolutely must get outside and get active.

Step #4: Give Your Brain a Mineral Boost

There are specific supplements that can improve mitochondrial functioning. One of the most important is magnesium, which many people are deficient in.

Magnesium is a critical mineral for the energy-producing enzymes in your mitochondria.

Now, you'll see lots of different types of magnesium supplements on the market. I recommend magnesium threonate, which, unlike other forms of magnesium, can penetrate the blood-brain barrier.

One good product is Neuro-Mag, which you can buy at **www.lifeextension.com.**

Step #5: Help Your Mitochondria Get the Most Out of Food

When you eat, energy-producing electrons are stripped out of food and delivered to your mitochondria. Two important supplements that help deliver those electrons are CoQ10 and PQQ.

You've probably heard a bit about how Coenzyme Q10 (CoQ10) is great for your heart, because it helps heart cells' mitochondria produce more energy. Well, it does the same thing for the mitochondria in your brain cells, too.

And PQQ, short for pyrroloquinoline quinone, provides essentially the same function by helping to deliver energy to mitochondria.

At **www.lifeextension.com** you can find a product called Super Ubiquinol CoQ10 with BioPQQ that provides both ingredients in one formula.

If my Brain Surge Protocol seems simple and straight-forward, that's because it is. Supporting your brain cells' mitochondria doesn't have to be difficult.

But taking these five steps, as my own patients will

tell you, can go a long way toward energizing your brain, reversing memory loss and keeping your mind razor sharp well into your golden years.

Bonus Content! Your Brain Cells Are Dying of Thirst... and You'll Never Believe Why

Remember how much better cell phones and wireless Internet were going to make our lives?

We'd have all the knowledge of the world at our fingertips, right? Well, it's become clear that lots of these technological wonders are harming our brains more than helping them.

You see, science is proving that the type of radiation produced by cell phones, microwaves, Wi-Fi and cell phone towers can wreak havoc on our mitochondria and our brains.

This radiation has been shown in many studies to cause psychiatric symptoms like anxiety, fatigue and depression.

So how is this happening? Well, we know that the radiation from our favorite electronic devices affects certain calcium channels in our nervous systems.

But, just as importantly, research has documented that exposure to electromagnetic fields can lead to the dehydration of cells.

That's a big problem, because water is a main power source for our mitochondria. And keeping our mitochondria healthy is essential to preserving our memories and normal brain function.

Unfortunately, these electromagnetic field are getting a lot harder to avoid... especially now that it seems like they're building a cell phone tower on every block.

That's why it's particularly important to make sure you're staying hydrated and drinking water throughout the day. Your brain cells might be a lot more dehydrated than you'd ever imagine.

[WARNING] COULD THIS DRUG ERASE YOUR MEMORY?

I've been practicing medicine for 35 years — and it doesn't have to be as complicated as some docs make it out to be.

In fact, I've always operated by a couple of really simple rules:

1. Never do anything that could make a patient worse.
2. If it's not a treatment I'd accept for myself, my wife, or my three sons, I'm sure as heck not going to recommend it to you…

But, believe it or not, common sense is in pretty short supply in the medical field today.

And if you're someone who gets up several times a night to pee, you may be learning that the hard way.

If you had to choose between an overactive bladder and dementia, which would you choose?

Stupid question, right?

I'll take a few extra trips to the bathroom over losing my mind any day of the year!

But would you believe that there are more than 7 MILLION people in the U.S. who are being asked to put their brains at risk, just so they can pee less at night?

That's about how many people are taking oxybutynin (Ditropan), a common drug prescribed to treat urinary problems. Multiple studies have linked this drug to thinking problems and an increased risk of dementia in older people, even with short-term use.

If that's not enough of a kick in the pants, it turns out this drug doesn't even work well in elderly patients!

Why would ANY doctor prescribe a drug with these known risks to seniors? I'll tell you why: MONEY and GOVERNMENT RED TAPE.

In fact, most Medicare Part D plans require patients to try oxybutynin — and have it fail — before they can try something else.

Am I the only one who finds that suspicious?

I don't want to make light of the quality of life issues tied to an overactive bladder. The need to urinate frequently — and urgently — can make you second-guess even a simple trip to the barber shop. And the potential for incontinence can be even more paralyzing.

But there are better solutions to this problem — ones that don't have you trading in your brain to keep your dignity.

I've found that a few simple lifestyle changes, as well as some targeted supplements, work wonders.

Two of my go-to supplements for bladder support are pygeum and saw palmetto. Both have a long history — and plenty of science — supporting their effectiveness in both bladder and prostate health.

But one of my favorite solutions is absolutely free: spend some time in the sun.

The underlying cause of an overactive bladder is inflammation, and one of the best ways to combat that is sunlight. The sun is the best source of vitamin D — something your body cannot produce on its own — and vitamin D plays a significant role in preventing chronic inflammation.

Now that's what I call smart medicine.

DEPRESSION'S SECRET CAUSE REVEALED

I'm sure I don't need to tell you that depression has practically become an epidemic… and we all know someone who has been affected.

According to a recent report, global depression rates have risen a whopping 20 percent over just the past decade.

There are 322 million people suffering from depression right now. That's roughly the population of the entire United States.

Alarming? Yes.

Shocking? Hardly.

The rising depression rates are something I've been warning about for years. And the cause is something that our government… and even lots of docs… don't want to talk about.

Our excessive exposure to artificial **blue light** is responsible for depression — and a host of other conditions, too.

Blue light is the kind caused by cell phones, computers, and flat screen televisions. And those "energy-efficient"

LED light bulbs that are supposed to be saving the planet are the worst offenders of all!

With today's technology-driven world, people are glued to blue-light emitting devices practically 24/7, and it's ruining our health.

When we are exposed to blue light constantly, it disrupts our bodies' natural clocks and circadian rhythms.

Our bodies basically can't tell night from day, and this throws our production of melatonin out of whack.

It would be impossible for me to overstress the importance of our circadian rhythm. This 24-hour clock releases hormones that regulate appetite, energy, mood, sleep, and more.

Even the slightest disruption in this critical life-cycle can wreak havoc on both our physical and emotional health. Just think about how something as simple as flying from one coast to the other can produce "jet lag" that can impact you for days.

One recent study showed that people who were exposed to chronic light at night started showing signs of depression after just a few weeks.

The constant exposure to blue light at the wrong time of day, and the subsequent disruption in circadian rhythms, are a recipe for health disaster — and it is definitely a factor in the rising rates of depression.

Before committing to a lifetime of (expensive, dangerous) antidepressants, wouldn't it make sense to tackle a potential cause? Especially one as simple as this?

That's what I call a no-brainer.

Here's what to do:

Short of avoiding all contact with electronics and going to bed when the sun goes down, the easiest, cheapest, most effective solution is to wear amber blue-light blocking glasses starting at 8 PM. You can pick them up at **www.amazon.com.**

You'll notice you'll get sleepy almost instantly. And over time, as you learn to follow your body's natural circadian rhythms, you'll notice you'll feel better too.

If you have money to burn, don't spend it on the drug Band-Aids that Big Pharma shoves down your throat. Spend it on a vacation. Pick up a hobby. Take your wife to a fancy dinner.

Live a little! Not only will it be a better use of your hard-earned money, it'll boost your spirits as well.

HERE'S MY WEIRD RECIPE FOR BRAIN POWER SUPERFOOD

Earlier in this chapter I talked about the importance of DHA for brain health, and how it helps power the mitochondria in our brain cells.

And there's a food I've been relying on for years to give my brain all the DHA it needs.

But I have to warn you — you're probably going to find it a little strange.

It's fish eggs or "roe." My favorite are salmon eggs.

Salmon eggs are a powerhouse of nutrition, containing most of the essential fat-soluble vitamins including vitamin A, vitamin D and vitamin K2. Salmon eggs also contain vital minerals including zinc and iodine.

But here's the best part…

Salmon eggs contain up to *3.5 times* the amount of DHA you'd get in salmon flesh.

Let me give you a little pointer on how you can make eating salmon eggs simple and possibly less expensive.

I buy my salmon roe frozen in a 1 kg. tray (you can get this at lots of seafood stores). I take the frozen eggs and a sturdy sharp knife, and while they still frozen, cut them into squares.

It's kind of like when you used to cut up those extremely toxic Rice Krispie treats when you were a kid.

I'll divide this 1 kg. tray of fish eggs into 20 sections. So I now have a portion of superfood for 20 days.

This is great for those days when you can't find fresh seafood, or your schedule is really hectic.

Once you cut the sections, place it all back in the freezer. To eat, just break off a serving and let it thaw either at room temperature or, if you are going to eat it the next day, let it thaw in the refrigerator overnight.

When making roe they add some salt. And to me salmon roe has a taste that is weird at first, but grows on you.

Getting enough DHA is extremely important for you, your kids, and even your grandkids. I've noticed toddlers love fish eggs and it makes a great finger food.

Some primitive cultures had an ancient knowledge or intuition about how important this food was. As an example, the famed researcher Weston Price wrote about how mountain natives in Peru would travel, sometimes hundreds of miles, to the coast and collect fish eggs. They would then dry the eggs and carry them back to the mountain villages.

Even though they didn't have the science, these cultures seemed to know that they felt healthier... and likely thought better... when fish eggs were part of their diet.

I've seen the same results with myself and my patients. So be adventurous and give fish eggs a try.

HAVE A CASE OF THE "BLAHS?" HERE'S WHAT TO DO

Lots of the patients I treat — especially seniors — don't have what I'd call full-blown depression.

Instead, they just feel crappy, fatigued, and like they've lost their zest for life.

Things they used to love, like knitting or bowling with friends, just don't seem to bring them any pleasure any more.

In other words, they have what I call a case of the "blahs."

If this sounds like you, I might have the answer you've been looking for.

I've found that low levels of dopamine — an essential neurotransmitter — are common, and practically an epidemic.

When present in normal levels, dopamine gives us a feeling of well-being.

Dopamine is also associated with the feeling of pleasure we get with certain activities. As we age, dopamine goes down and often a person's pleasure in life goes down along with it.

Dopamine levels start decreasing generally after the age of 45, and when dopamine levels are low there's accelerated brain aging.

So what can you do to get your dopamine levels up to snuff?

Well, studies show that when the enzyme MAO-B increases in your body, your dopamine levels decrease.

There are drugs on the market that block MAO-B, but you don't need to resort to that.

Recently, there's been a supplement that's been shown to inhibit MAO-B. It's called wild green oat extract.

This supplement has been shown to increase some aspects of cognitive function, brain processing speed, and mood. One good wild green oat extract product is Life Extension's Dopa-Mind, which you can pick up at **www.lifeextension.com.**

Is also been discovered that dopamine production is increased with exposure to light in the eye. That means spending time in the sun each day — without those UV-blocking sunglasses.

Try combining sun exposure with supplementation, and there's a good chance you're going to finally leave that case of the "blahs" behind you for good.

IS THIS "HEALTHY" SWEETENER POISONING YOUR BRAIN?

It's in some of the most popular chewing gums and diet drinks today.

I'm talking about aspartame, that no-calorie sweetener that was supposed to be healthy and help us keep our waistlines in check.

But if aspartame is a big part of your diet, there's an urgent warning you need to hear.

There's a good chance you're poisoning your brain!

This artificial sweetener was approved for use in 1981 in the United States.

Since the introduction of aspartame, Alzheimer's disease deaths have increased 100 times and autism incidence has increased 25 times.

Other diseases that have dramatically increased including lupus, multiple sclerosis and many types of cancers.

A pharmaceutical company created aspartame and got it approved for use in food. And, sure enough, it's the drug companies that are benefiting the most from the spikes in diseases.

Now, if you're like some of my patients, you might say, "I'm tired of these conspiracy theories, Dr. G. If aspartame was really that bad, science would have figured it out by now."

Well, science did figure it out a long time ago. Our government is just too chicken to take action.

I highly suggest you check out a book by Dr. Woodrow Montes, an emeritus professor at Arizona State University, called *While Science Sleeps — A Sweetener Kills.*

It contains convincing evidence that methanol, which is a poisonous substance that's hidden in aspartame, is converted in the body to formaldehyde. And formaldehyde is absolutely toxic to your brain and other organs.

This book is very scientifically grounded with thousands of references. And once you read it, you'll never touch aspartame again.

My advice? Read every label. Don't buy any soft drinks, chewing gum, food, or any other product that contains aspartame, NutraSweet, Equal, Spoonful or Equal Measure (aspartame under disguised names). The evidence of toxicity is overwhelming.

UNCLE SAM DECLARING WAR ON THIS VITAL BRAIN HORMONE

By now you know that I believe that hormonal changes — and disruptions — are a major contributor to chronic diseases, including those that affect the brain.

And if you want to keep a healthy brain — and live the long, disease-free life you deserve — there's one hormone that's absolutely essential.

It's called dehydroepiandrosterone, or DHEA for short.

DHEA is a wonder hormone that can reverse the effects of aging and have you thinking better and more clearly than ever.

So why is our government trying to take this powerful natural cure away from you?

Things got awfully dicey in 2007, when a bill was before Congress to have DHEA's status changed to an anabolic steroid. That would have made it basically an illegal substance.

Thankfully, this law wasn't passed — but Big Pharma isn't going to give up its efforts to get DHEA off the market.

Powerful drug company lobbyists and the government

have a vested interest in keeping alternative health remedies out of your hands, so you have to rely on prescription meds instead.

And DHEA is one of the most powerful, natural brain-boosting remedies around.

To give you some background, DHEA levels usually drop quickly after the age of 50, so you are more likely to have low levels and benefit from supplementing if you are older.

Levels decline 75 percent to 80 percent by the time we reach age 70.

And DHEA plays a major role in brain function as we age. Studies show that supplementation can improve both memory and decision making.

Low levels of DHEA have been associated with depression, and supplementing has been shown to improve symptoms.

A National Institutes of Mental Health study on DHEA to treat depression stated, "We find DHEA to be effective treatment for midlife-onset major and minor depression."

Has your psychiatrist or doctor who prescribes your antidepressant ever told you that?

And the health benefits of DHEA go far beyond our brains.

DHEA also helps your bones and joints. Randomized trials have shown improvements in bone density, and that DHEA might prevent arthritis.

This hormone also keeps your immune system from overreacting by reducing allergies and inflammatory cytokines that contribute to autoimmune diseases.

Low DHEA levels have been shown to raise the risk of diabetes, heart disease and obesity. One mechanism for this may be that high DHEA levels reduce abdominal fat, which I know is music to lots of my patients' ears.

Other studies have shown that DHEA helps sex drive in both men and women and it also causes youthful changes in the skin.

If you're at risk for any of the above conditions, particularly if you have been placed on drugs for any of these, here's what you should do.

First off, I don't believe anyone should take DHEA without first measuring their blood levels.

The test is simple and performed by most labs. Just ask your doctor to run the DHEA-S level.

The normal range varies with age but the ideal range you'll be shooting for is 300–490 ug/dl in men and 250–400 ug/dl in women.

Women should not take DHEA if they have an estrogen-dependent cancer and men should not take it if they have prostate cancer.

An average dose might be 12.5 mg a day for women and 12.5–50 mg a day for men. DHEA can be given in pills or capsules that you swallow — but that has the downside of being metabolized in the liver before going to your body.

A better way is through the skin in a transdermal preparation or tablets that dissolve in your mouth (you can buy dissolvable DHEA tablets at **www.lifeextension.com**). That way, the DHEA reaches your bloodstream before going to the liver.

The Life Extension product is ½ to 1 tablet of the 25 mg of DHEA each day.

After you have been on DHEA for two months, it is important to check the levels of DHEA-S again and see where you are. I usually shoot for getting the blood levels into the top quartile of the normal range. I don't recommend getting your levels above the normal range.

CHAPTER TWO

THE DOCTOR'S SECRET TO LIMITLESS ENERGY

IS THIS UNDIAGNOSED DISORDER LEAVING YOU EXHAUSTED?

I have a confession to make.

When it comes to energy levels, I've never had much of a problem. I've hiked the Grand Canyon… run marathons… climbed some of the high peaks of the Himalayas… and carried elk meat on my back for miles.

I've been pushing my body (sometimes against my better judgment) to the limit for years.

But I regularly see patients who are my age or younger, who aren't so lucky.

They shuffle into my office looking tired, worn out, and in pain.

They look 10 years older than they are — and they feel even worse!

And, unfortunately, many of these patients have one thing in common.

They've been complaining about their energy levels to their doctors for years — and they've never been given a good explanation for why they're exhausted and what to do about it.

And the problem has gotten a lot worse since prescription antidepressants hit the market. Lots of docs will just take the easy (and lazy) way out, and throw you on a happy pill like Prozac and see if it makes a difference.

Well, good luck with that.

The truth is, there may be a very simple and logical reason your energy levels are in the tank. And fixing the problem can get you surging with energy like you haven't felt in years.

It all starts with…

An energy-sapping disorder that most doctors NEVER diagnose!

I'm talking about adrenal fatigue. And it's practically becoming an epidemic, even though most mainstream doctors have been slow to accept it.

The adrenals are located on top of your kidneys, and when they're over-worked they can start to wear down and leave you exhausted.

When your adrenals stop working entirely, you have something called Addison's disease. You might remember that President John F. Kennedy suffered from this.

For most people, it doesn't go that far… but under-performing adrenals can still throw your energy levels into a tailspin.

The adrenal glands make important hormones that help us with stress. The one that is secreted during sudden stress is adrenalin (epinephrine).

This hormone gets us ready to fight or run. It raises the blood pressure, dilates the pupils, and opens the arteries to the large muscles.

Another hormone produced in the adrenals that is increased with stress is cortisol. Cortisol mobilizes stored energy so that it can be used.

Now, here's where things get tricky…

When I see a patient with early stress, they will tend to have elevated cortisol levels.

But when a person has been dealing with chronic, long-term stress, their cortisol levels may be extremely low.

In other words, the hormone production in their adrenals has begun to peter out, leaving their energy levels sinking like a stone.

In fact...

Low cortisol levels are a MAJOR sign of adrenal fatigue.

So what are some of the other telltale signs of adrenal fatigue? The major ones include:

- Difficulty getting up in the morning;
- Continuing fatigue despite adequate sleep;
- Craving for salt or salty foods;
- Lack of energy and increased effort to do daily tasks;
- Decreased sex drive;
- An increased inability to handle stress;
- Longer recovery time from illnesses or trauma;
- Low blood pressure;
- Light-headedness when standing up quickly;
- Irritability or depressed mood;
- An increase in allergies; and
- Lack of mental clarity and memory.

When I'm diagnosing adrenal fatigue, I'll look for these symptoms and look for other signs, like low cortisol levels. It's amazing to me how many people have never been properly tested for this disorder.

The good news is that once adrenal fatigue is diagnosed, you can start working to give your adrenals the support they need. And in just weeks you can start to notice...

A HUGE energy surge as your adrenals kick back into action!

First, there are some key nutrients that are needed in the production of the adrenal hormones. These include vitamin C, vitamin E, magnesium, pantothenic acid, niacin, and vitamin B6.

The good news? You can find most of these nutrients in a quality multivitamin, which you can pick up just about anywhere.

For example, Life Force by Source Naturals has all of these ingredients, and you can pick it up for less than $30 a month at **www.vitacost.com.**

Second, I recommend that patients add an "adaptogen" such as ashwagandha to their supplement regimens.

Adaptogens are natural remedies that help regulate stress and stabilize hormone production throughout your body. And ashwagandha, an Indian herb, is one of the most powerful and effective adaptogens around.

I've seen patients taking ashwagandha who report feeling more relaxed, more energized, and are able to think more clearly in just days!

You can pick up NOW Foods ashwagandha extract at **www.puritan.com.**

Now, of course, there are some mainstream prescription treatments out there — and you probably want to avoid them the way a cat avoids a bath.

In the old days, adrenal glandular preparations from animals were popular for treating people with adrenal fatigue, but when the corticosteroid drugs came on the market they went out of favor.

The problem is that corticosteroid drugs come with serious side effects, like high blood pressure, thinning bones, and even glaucoma! Why take those risks?

The other option is to use prescription cortisol. The

problem with this is you are replacing only one of several adrenal hormones so it is not as likely to be all that effective.

It's a Band-Aid… and not a great one.

One word of caution for both you and your doctor.

It is common for adrenal problems to coexist with thyroid problems. I have found that if you try and correct the thyroid when a person has underlying adrenal fatigue, the thyroid symptoms will often get worse with treatment.

So if you've ever had a thyroid treatment that failed, this could be a major clue.

Unfortunately, adrenal fatigue isn't on the radar for lots of doctors. If you feel you are experiencing the symptoms I've discussed, you must be proactive and find a qualified natural medicine doctor who will guide you through the process of diagnosis and treatment.

The American College for Advancement in Medicine has a physician finder on its website that is a great place to start. Just go to **www.acam.org** and click the "Resources" tab.

THE TECHNOLOGY THAT'S DESTROYING YOUR ENERGY (AND YOUR HEALTH)

We're all familiar with the concept of the canary in the coal mine, right?

That was when miners would take an extremely sensitive animal, like a canary, down into the mine with them.

And while they were working, they would periodically look over at the canary and make sure it was alive. Because if it had fallen off its perch, that means you better run like heck to get out of the tunnel because methane or carbon monoxide levels are rising and you'll soon be dead.

Well, I believe we have a similar situation in modern medicine today. But the "canaries" we're talking about aren't super-sensitive birds… they're super-sensitive people!

You may be one of them — and this could explain your fatigue and lots of other health problems.

These super-sensitive people come into my office all the time, and generally their health is going down the tubes fast.

They're commonly suffering from crippling fatigue, but it doesn't stop there. They also may have irritable bowel syndrome, migraine headaches, chronic pain, insomnia, depression, weight gain, and brain fog.

Sometimes they've even developed chronic, horrible diseases like autoimmune disorders, diabetes, heart disease, cancer, chronic infections, Alzheimer's disease or other neurological conditions.

The first step toward healing these patients is asking them...

The ONE question that could change your life... and *reverse* your failing health!

Here's the question: Do you feel significantly better when you get out in the middle of nowhere, like out in the wilderness?

If you haven't experimented with this, give it a try as soon as possible.

When patients answer yes (and lots of them do), I recommend a thorough evaluation of their exposure to electromagnetic fields or EMFs. These EMFs can absolutely destroy your health, and I'll explain how in a moment.

I look for three kinds of possible exposures, such as magnetic fields (which are measured in milligauss); electric fields (which are measured in volts on the skin); and radiofrequency/microwave (which are measured in microwatts/cm²).

So what are the sources of these fields? The most common ones are computers, tablets like the iPad, and smartphones. The wireless devices are usually the worst.

Cordless phones cause exposure, as do cell phone towers. Other sources are power lines, in-home electrical wiring, microwave ovens, televisions, refrigerators, lighting and other electrical equipment. In other words...

The technology that's supposed to improve our lives is making us sick!

So how exactly do these EMF exposures harm us?

Animal and human studies have shown evidence of cancer

risk and that EMFs cause disruption in hormone levels and other bodily functions.

Our bodies, and thus our cells, are in tune with the Earth's magnetic field called the Shuman field. The theory is that our cells operate by a circadian clock, even on the molecular level, and that depends on Earth's electromagnetic field.

These competing magnetic fields (from EMFs) may mess up our sensing of these natural fields and thus cause cellular dysfunction. This would logically result in a multitude of health problems that we see.

It is also interesting to see our health problems skyrocket as these interfering fields have become more common. Sure this is circumstantial, but I see evidence of it all the time.

I know this is a hard pill for most of us to swallow. With industry and government introducing more and more of these devices and these fields, most of us have become completely addicted to our gadgets, and won't give them up until they drop our body in a casket.

Yes, this is an inconvenient truth, but a truth nevertheless.

Another question you may be asking is, "Do I want to wait until the government sets reasonable standards and does the safety testing?"

When there are trillions of dollars at stake both in the government and in industry, you can be sure no good studies are going to come out about the harm that these electromagnetic fields are causing, at least not until the body count is very high.

If you search for it, you can find plenty of evidence that these EMFs are harmful to life and I come to that conclusion from my anecdotal experience with patients for over 30 years and after reviewing the research that is available.

These EMFs significantly affect health and I believe it's just a matter of time, because of their constant increase, that there will eventually be a health catastrophe.

My advice to you is to take advantage of my super-sensitive, canary-like patients. They are telling us, "run for your life." There are some common-sense ways to limit your EMF exposure, including:

- Using a standard phone with a chord in your home;
- Keep all electronic devices out of your bed-room at night. This will give you 8 hours of limited or no EMF exposure a day;
- Set your wireless router on a Christmas light timer, so it's off at night;
- Keep your cell phone on airplane mode as much as possible;
- Use an ethernet cable instead of Wi-Fi on your computer.

I can't tell you the number of patients I've had who have seen their energy levels restored — and their health improved — after taking small steps like these. I hope you or someone you love will be next.

THE "FINGERPRINTS OF GOD" PROTOCOL TURNS YOUR CELLS INTO ENERGY POWERHOUSES

Remember how you were going to spend your retirement years doing all the things you love?

You were going to hit the golf links a couple of times a week… and maybe finally expand that garden.

But, lately, just getting off the couch feels like a chore.

Your energy levels are in the tank and you can feel your health and vigor slipping away.

Well, you don't have to live the rest of your life that way. Because I'm going to show you how to boost your energy levels and ward off chronic disease all at the same time. And it all starts with a very simple premise.

The secret to unlimited energy (and good health) starts with your cells!

In particular, I'm talking about your mitochondria, which are like your cells' powerhouses.

And if your mitochondria aren't in good shape, everything else you try to improve your health is going to feel like rowing a boat upstream.

Now, you may remember from school that mitochondria

direct the energy production for our cells.

But we're learning that there's much more to mitochondria than that. In fact...

Your mitochondria are like the "fingerprints of God!"

You see, scientists have studied the composition of mitochondria, and discovered something amazing.

They're not really human in origin. In fact, they have their own DNA.

But they're responsible for nearly all of life's processes... we can't live or function without them.

They're like these divine "batteries" placed inside our bodies that give us energy and make all of our biological systems work.

So how do they do that? Basically, they take electrons from our food and transport them, like an electrical cable, to form a proton flow across the mitochondrial membrane.

This energy flow helps activate something called ATP, which is a main energy source for our cells and powers most of our bodies' functions.

So keeping your mitochondria healthy produces a strong supply of energy you can feel — and that will fight fatigue.

But mitochondria also generate the energy our organs need to function right.

Studies tell us that defective and deficient numbers of mitochondria are connected to virtually all degenerative diseases, particularly:

- Diabetes;
- Alzheimer's disease;
- Cancer; and
- Congestive heart failure.

And these are ALL increasing. Scientists have discovered that mitochondria become damaged with aging. A study looking at the mitochondria of five-year-olds showed that the mitochondria had near-perfect structure and function.

But when they tested a 90-year-old person, 95 percent of the mitochondria were damaged.

So what can we do to improve our mitochondrial health, boost our energy levels, and restore our health?

You can start with these 7 steps (and many of them won't cost a dime):

1. Eat foods that are rich in electrons, such as healthy fats and fish. Your body actually strips the electrons from this food and delivers them to your mitochondria.

2. Drink unfluoridated water. You can buy a water filter if your community fluoridates water. Believe it or not, fluoride actually blocks the transfer of electrical charges in our cells. That's not something you'll ever hear from all those dental groups pushing fluoridation.

3. Avoid bromide, which is a halogen like fluoride. It's found in processed grains and in hot tub and pool cleaning chemicals.

4. Maintain a diverse microflora in your gut. This helps with the energy transfer from your food to your mitochondria. Taking a daily probiotic is an easy way to keep your gut bacteria healthy.

5. Try spending several minutes a day on deep breathing or meditation, to increase your oxygen flow. Oxygen is essential to the transfer of electrons to your cells. Did you ever wonder why folks who meditate or practice deep breathing seem to be teeming with energy?

6. Decrease any exposure to non-native electromagnetic fields (EMFs), like you get from computers, tablets, smart phones, and other electronic devices. For more, see **The Technology That's DESTROYING Your Energy (And Your Health)** earlier in this chapter.
7. Begin supplementing with pyrroloquinoline quinone (VitalinQ), or PQQ for short. PQQ is a recently discovered substance, found in most fruits and vegetables, and it's absolutely essential to mitochondrial health.

When animals are deprived of PQQ, they have stunted growth and abundant problems and these problems are reversed when PQQ is put back into the diet.

You see, the PQQ molecule is involved in electron transfer in the mitochondria and has the advantage of being an extremely stable molecule.

Experimentally it's been shown to stimulate the growth of **brand new mitochondria** through activation of key genes. And the more new, healthy mitochondria you grow, the better you're going to feel — I guarantee it.

But the wonders of PQQ don't end there.

It's also been shown to safeguard a gene whose malfunction has been related to an early step in the development of Parkinson's disease.

Studies have shown that PQQ limits brain damage in stroke and heart attack in animal models. Other studies show it prevents the formation of amyloid beta structures which are involved in Alzheimer's disease.

Studies have been done supplementing PQQ in humans and showing improved cognitive function in middle age people.

As I said, you can get PQQ from fruits and vegetables

— but to get a really concentrated dose, supplementing is a smart idea.

You can buy PQQ caps from the Life Extension Foundation at **www.lifeextension.com.** It comes with a purified, highly potent form of PQQ, which is what you should look for.

Also, studies have also shown that you can enhance the effects of PQQ when you also take CoQ10 (ubiquinone) supplements. CoQ10 is also proven to support your mito-chondria and help generate more cellular energy.

You can purchase CoQ10 supplements online or at just about any vitamin shop. It's becoming a very popular supplement.

Remember to combine PQQ and CoQ10 with the other elements of my protocol. By doing these things in concert, you'll get the best results for your mitochondria.

CHAPTER THREE

CANCER-CONQUERING SECRETS FROM THE MEDICAL UNDERGROUND

REVOLUTIONARY TREATMENT CURES PROSTATE CANCER WITHOUT SIDE EFFECTS

If you've ever been diagnosed with prostate cancer, you know how quickly the news can go from bad to worse.

First there's that frightening diagnosis... the moment that you realize there's been a tumor growing inside of you. Then, you learn about the barbaric treatments that mainstream medicine is offering.

I call them the Big 3 — surgery, radiation, and chemotherapy. And lots of guys have learned the hard way that they can leave you incontinent or even wreck your sex life forever.

Well, there's another option out there — one that could save your life and your quality of life. It's safe, comes without side effects, and has **an impressive 90 percent success rate.**

It's called hyperthermia, and if you haven't heard of it, there's a good reason.

Our government has practically declared war on this cancer breakthrough, and is doing everything it can to keep it away from guys like you.

Meet Tony (He Just Might Save Your Life)

When my patient, Tony, came to me for his yearly checkup, his prostate specific antigen (PSA) was double the limit of the normal range.

Now, the PSA is pretty controversial and the U.S. Preventive Services Task Force has not recommend routine PSA screening since 2008. That's mostly because PSA screening often leads to unnecessary biopsies and overtreatment.

But I'll be honest with you — anytime one of my patients has a PSA that's double what it should be, I get concerned. So I sent him to a urologist for an MRI (See "Why MRIs Run Circles Around Biopsies" on page 51).

That's when we got the bad news — Tony had aggressive prostate cancer, although, fortunately, it was confined to his prostate.

And, like lots of guys with aggressive prostate cancer, Tony was given two options — dangerous radiation to kill the prostate cancer cells (which has been shown to promote the growth of new cancers) and a radical prostatectomy where they remove the prostate surgically.

I was disappointed but not shocked that Tony was never given hyperthermia as a treatment option. More than 176,000 American men a year are diagnosed with prostate cancer, and almost none of them are told about hyperthermia.

That's when I educated Tony about this revolutionary treatment and a clinic in Germany that's changing and saving men's' lives. And they may be able to do the same for you or someone you love.

A Cancer Cure Without Side Effects

About 10 years ago, I attended a lecture by an oncologist from Germany who presented 100 cases of prostate cancer patients treated with hyperthermia.

The science behind hyperthermia is incredibly straight-forward. A simple catheter is passed through your urinary tract into your bladder and it heats your prostate for a period of two hours.

You see, prostate cancer cells are more sensitive to heat than normal cells. The heat can kill cancer cells and leave the normal cells unharmed.

Now, I know most guys like to avoid catheters the way a dog avoids a bath — but trust me, it's a whole lot better than having your prostate cut out.

And here's the best part — the treatment has a 90 percent success rate with virtually NO side effects after treatment!

When I checked for Tony, I found that the Klinik St. Georg in Aibling, Germany was continuing to offer hyper-thermia for prostate cancer. And now going on 20 years, they still have that same, glowing 90 percent success rate.

But most urologists in America are still refusing to adopt the treatment, despite how well (and safely) it works. In fact, there's plenty of evidence that mainstream medicine and the federal government have been conspiring for years to keep hyperthermia out of your hands.

Our Government's Secret Fight Against Hyperthermia

When I first met that German oncologist a decade ago, he shared a story that ought to have thousands of guys storming Washington, D.C.

He told me that he actually presented his data to the Food and Drug Administration on the 100 patients treated with hyperthermia. He proved that the treatment had a 90 percent success rate and no side effects.

The FDA shot it down right away.

And if you're wondering why a simple, effective, safe procedure is not being allowed, let me solve the mystery for you. It's all about money.

It appears to me that the FDA is protecting the current treatment model. There are many vested interests that want to keep the $50,000+ prostatectomies going.

Hospitals are spending upwards of $2 million on surgical robots, like the daVinci. And you'd best believe they're serious about recovering that investment.

The FDA doesn't want to ruffle any financial feathers of these established treatments, even though there's no evidence that they are more effective than doing nothing, as far as mortality is concerned.

Plus, urologists and surgeons understand the psyche of the typical American man. When most guys learn they have cancer, their aggressive sides kick in — they just want that sucker out. So the mainstream often has little trouble steering men to potentially dangerous (and often life-wrecking) treatments.

How to Handle a Prostate Cancer Diagnosis

When you're diagnosed with prostate cancer, don't let anyone rush you into a treatment decision.

Believe it or not, springing into action at light speed isn't always as important as some urologists will make it sound.

There was a major clinical trial called PROTECT that did a 10-year follow-up on guys with prostate cancer that included active surveillance (where you essentially monitor your prostate cancer to see if it gets worse and needs treatment), radical prostatectomy and radiation.

There was no difference in survival between the three groups. Absolutely none.

Remember that the next time someone wants to wheel you in for surgery before you've had a chance to catch your breath.

Instead, take time to consider your options.

If you're up for a medical vacation, you can learn more about Klinik St. Georg at **www.klinik-st-georg.de/**. The website is in German, but most Internet browsers (like Google Chrome) will translate it for you, and you'll find staff who speak perfect English.

Another treatment that's actually available in the USA is cryotherapy, which freezes prostate cancer cells. It has far fewer side effects than surgery, and seems to get good results.

Remember, too, that simple lifestyle changes can have a big effect on prostate cancer.

Food and supplements that have shown to curb the development of prostate cancer include the cruciferous vegetables (cabbage, cauliflower, broccoli, Brussels sprouts), as well as lycopene, saw palmetto, and beta sitosterol.

Lycopene, saw palmetto, and beta sitosterol are all sold as stand-alone supplements and in combination in several multi-ingredient prostate supplements.

Finally, it's important to fix any circadian disruptions in your life (the day and night cycle). Studies show that men who hide from the sun double their risk for prostate cancer. Low melatonin levels, which is a consequence of artificial light at night, have also been shown to significantly increase prostate cancer risk.

If you are diagnosed with prostate cancer, take a deep breath. There is no reason to rush your decision on what to do next. Get a second, and even third, opinion. And don't be afraid to consider a medical vacation overseas.

Bonus Content! Why MRIs Run Circles Around Biopsies

When your PSA levels start creeping up, the first thing many urologists want to do is send you for a biopsy.

But before you sign on for this painful — and often unnecessary procedure — you need to know that you have other options.

New research just published from the PROMIS study shows that magnetic resonance imaging (MRI) is twice as sensitive as a biopsy for detecting aggressive prostate cancer. Better still, it's pain-free and comes without the risks of biopsies.

THIS "NUTRIENT 8" TREATMENT DESTROYS CANCER CELLS

Imagine sitting with your doctor in his office… huge smiles of relief on both of your faces.

Your latest imaging results are back. And they've proven, again, that your tumor is continuing to shrink.

It's literally melting away. And you haven't had a single chemo drip or sat for any radiation sessions.

People just like you are getting these results — and they're using an alternative cancer treatment that many patients are never told about.

It's called intravenous vitamin C (IVC), and the mainstream has been trying to blacklist it for years.

Fortunately, the tide is starting to turn a bit.

You see, Nobel Prize winner Linus Pauling first proposed using vitamin C to treat cancer decades ago. People called him a quack at the time — but now we know that he had discovered something revolutionary.

That's because he understood that at high enough doses, vitamin C produces hydrogen peroxide in our bodies — and that is toxic to cancer cells.

In fact, researchers have proven that IVC actually attacks cancer through eight different pathways, which is why some call it "Nutrient 8."

Of course, mainstream doctors and drug companies did everything they could to try to convince the public that Pauling was wrong... and crazy.

But we know now that he was absolutely right.

Numerous studies have now proven the cancer-killing ability of IVC, and it's used by alternative health doctors all across the country.

The University of Kansas Medical Center has developed a treatment protocol for doctors, and even the federal government has funded studies on it.

In one case, reported by federal health agencies, a 51-year-old woman with metastatic kidney cancer opted for IVC treatment. After just 7 months of twice-weekly infusions, her tumors had shrunk so dramatically that they were practically invisible on film!

In another case, a man with bladder cancer that was already spreading started getting IVC. He was completely cured — and when researchers checked in with him 9 years later, he was still in fantastic health.

What makes IVC so special as a cancer treatment is that it's incredibly versatile. In fact, a 2015 lab study out of Cornell found that it can even kill colorectal cancer cells with a genetic mutation that makes them hard to treat.

Of course, chemotherapy, surgery, and radiation are massive, multi-billion dollar industries. So many patients are never given the option of IVC.

If you want to give IVC a try, your best bet is to call alternative doctors in your market. The American College for Advancement in Medicine has a great physician locator at **www.acam.org** (look under the Resources tab).

You probably won't have to make too many calls before you

find a doctor who offers it — or knows someone who does.

Make sure you ask how long the doctor has been offering the treatment, and what his success rate has been. You always want to choose an experienced doctor you feel comfortable with.

If you're currently undergoing chemo, you should know that IVC has also been found to decrease side effects like fatigue and nausea. Any doctor can order up IVC, so talk to your doc about incorporating it into your treatment.

THIS WORLD WAR II SCIENTIST FOUND A RADICAL WAY TO BEAT CANCER

Maybe the only thing worse than a cancer diagnosis is how we treat the disease.

I've seen so many people over the years (and I bet you have, too), who have had their lives destroyed by poisonous mainstream treatments like radiation, chemotherapy, and surgery.

But what if there is a simpler... and safer... way to beat cancer? One that's been staring us in the face for more than 75 years?

It all comes down to an incredibly simple premise...

Starve cancer cells and they'll die — by the MILLIONS!

And, believe it or not, we have an old World War II scientist to thank for this breakthrough.

His name was Dr. Otto Warburg, and he was a German researcher who actually won the Nobel Prize in medicine in 1931.

He even continued his medical research during the war... under the direct approval of Adolf Hitler... which didn't win him too many fans.

But the fact is, Warburg was on to something HUGE.

He began by examining mitochondria — the tiny biological "batteries" that provide energy within each cell.

Mitochondria usually use oxygen to break down protein, fats and carbohydrates into energy.

When they are damaged or deprived of oxygen, they start breaking down sugar via fermentation. This inefficient process leads the half-starved cell to make "mistakes," including reproducing wildly — in other words, becoming cancerous.

In other words, sugar triggers everything. Even the mainstream admits cancer loves sugar.

In fact, to locate tumors within the body, physicians give patients pure glucose linked to a radioactive dye.

Cancer cells, hungry for glucose, gobble it up.

So could depriving cancer cells of glucose actually shrink or kill tumors?

Well, Warburg never got that far — but some modern researchers did.

To test the "Warburg Hypothesis," a Johns Hopkins researcher injected 19 cancerous rats with a compound called 3-bromopyruvate.

It "shuts the gate" on sugar's ability to enter cancerous cells.

All of the rats were cured and went on to have normal life spans.

Other animal studies, meanwhile, have shown that radically low-carbohydrate diets reduce tumor growth and improve survival in many types of cancer, including malignant glioma and cancer of the colon, GI tract and prostate.

There's still plenty of research ongoing. But if you or someone you love is suffering from cancer, a dramatically low-carb diet may be worth trying.

Because we already know that cancer loves sugar — and

with each passing decade, more and more evidence is surfacing that Warburg was right.

SHOULD YOU GET A PSA TEST? YOU MIGHT BE SURPRISED...

If there's one test that's leaving MILLIONS of men confused, it's prostate-specific antigen (PSA) screening.

We've heard that the PSA test is crucial for detecting prostate cancer early, and that it can save lives.

But lately the PSA has been getting some bad press, with even the government and the mainstream medical establishment coming out against it.

However, there are forces at work here that are more concerned with money than your good health.

And I still regularly recommend PSA testing to my patients — with a couple of big caveats.

You see, the United States Preventive Services Task Force recently decided that men should no longer get regular PSA testing to screen for prostate cancer. They say it can lead to overtreatment (which it can... more on that in a moment).

But is eliminating PSA testing really a good idea — or is this task force on a mission to reduce health care costs among seniors?

It's no secret that programs like Medicare and Medicaid

are going bust as health care costs skyrocket. And I'm pretty sure that when we're all dead, our health care costs for Uncle Sam are zero.

Accord to this Task Force, PSA testing has not been documented to save lives, so therefore, shouldn't be done. And I agree — to a point.

When PSA testing is used as a justification to overtreat you — to poke holes in your prostate and rip your prostate out of your body — then I agree it's not very valuable.

But because of the mainstream's obsession with overtreatment...

They're literally throwing out the baby with the bath water!

The fact is, PSA can be a marker that you are developing the conditions that may lead to prostate cancer and its spread. That's the truth.

Most doctors (even urologists) don't know that PSA functions as an enzyme to break down the natural barriers that surround cells called the extracellular matrix.

A high PSA is like a canary in the coal mine.

So by lowering PSA you may prevent any prostate cancer cells that are present from growing and spreading. In nixing the PSA the task force really shows they're not into prevention, and really don't even consider it.

The real lesson here is that by lowering your PSA, you can protect your extracellular matrix and keep a possible case of cancer from spreading.

In my experience, PSA is easy to reduce. Of course, Big Pharma has drugs like Avodart that come with a high cost and side effects.

But we really don't need these medications if you're willing to do an aggressive program of detoxification, nutrition and appropriate supplementation.

A list of nutrients, backed by decades of research, that

may help reduce PSA include:

- Boron;
- Milk thistle;
- Curcumin;
- Lycopene;
- Vitamin D; and
- Selenium.

You can pick up any of these supplements affordably at websites like **www.iherb.com** or **www.puritan.com.**

I also recommend you talk to your doctor about being tested for heavy metals. Studies have shown much higher levels of toxins, especially heavy metals, in cancerous prostates.

My recommendation is to test the PSA. If you have a PSA above 1, that's a "shot across the bow," and you should start taking the steps I've described to lower it.

That makes a lot more sense than just watching your PSA go up until it's time for a biopsy or prostatectomy.

And no matter what your PSA number, never rush into a surgery or other treatment plan. Always get multiple opinions and see if lowering your PSA naturally can help. That way you're protecting yourself against becoming a victim of overtreatment.

IS THIS WEED KILLER CANCER IN A BOTTLE?

Every time I see it, I shake my head in disbelief.

You can't walk into a Home Depot these days without seeing a gigantic stack of weed killers, positioned like an impulse buy.

It's kind of like in Wal-Mart where they have candy bars right next to checkout.

And, more often than not, these retailers are pushing bottles of Roundup, one of the most dangerous weed killers around.

Or, as I like to call it… cancer in a bottle.

Roundup is made by the major biotech company, Monsanto. And a major international health group — after years of research and over the objections of Monsanto — has declared that it's a likely cause of cancer.

But avoiding Roundup — and its main ingredient glyphosate — isn't as simple as skipping a purchase and keeping it off your garden or lawn.

Because these days, this dangerous weed killer is all over our food!

You see, many of our crops today have been genetically modified GMO to tolerate herbicides like Roundup.

But now weeds are becoming resistant to it, and farmers are using higher and higher amounts in an attempt to control weeds.

In America we use over 185 million pounds a year of Roundup. This is good for Monsanto, but not good for us.

What is the EPA doing to protect this from this growing threat? Well, they're simply increasing the amount of Roundup they'll let you eat.

Not too long ago, they upped the allowable limits for the amount of glyphosate that can remain on our food. In fact, the amounts they're now permitting go way above the dose that caused health problems in recent studies.

How short-sighted can you get?

Recent research has shown that glyphosate inhibits something called the P 450 enzyme system. This is a major system our body uses to detoxify chemicals that we're exposed to.

When animal studies of glyphosate are done over the entire lifespan of the animal, the chemical caused kidney and liver problems, greatly increased cancer risk, and led to a shorter lifespan.

I don't know about you... but none of that sounds too good to me.

The Roundup that many of us spray on the weeds that grow in the cracks in our driveways and in our lawns reduces our ability to get rid of all the other thousands of chemicals were exposed to. This leads to the chronic diseases that are increasing, including gastrointestinal disorders, obesity, diabetes, heart disease, depression, autism, infertility, cancer and Alzheimer's disease.

So what do I recommend? First, resist the temptation to buy a bottle of Roundup. If you buy this product, you're just encouraging them to make more to re-stock the shelves.

The second thing is to avoid any GMO containing foods. By switching to organic you avoid GMO herbicides like Roundup.

Organic produce may cost a bit more. But in the long run, your health is worth it.

Talk to most mainstream docs about how to prevent diseases,

THE BLISSFUL WAY
TO DETOX
(AND STOP CANCER)

and they'll either want you eating like a monk or working out like a Navy SEAL.

But what if I told there was a simple and safe way to prevent most of the common diseases that plague us — even cancer.

It's inexpensive, enjoyable, and you can do it from home — but your doctor probably doesn't know anything about it.

I'm talking about sauna treatments. And in addition to being a wonderful way to relax, science is showing that saunas can be powerful disease fighters.

Let me explain.

Earlier in this chapter, I told you about hyperthermia — a process that raises the temperatures of cancer cells to kill them.

That's because cancer cells don't tolerate extra heat as well as normal, healthy cells. So researchers found that you can heat up the body and kill cancer cells without killing healthy cells.

But this "heat as medicine" philosophy goes well beyond

cancer.

Another treatment rarely used is when a person has an infection that antibiotics won't touch. Doctors can inject a pyrogen (that's a fever inducing substance) and it can cure the infection where nothing else worked.

After all, a fever is your body's natural way of using heat to kill off foreign infections and invaders.

Excess heat also causes the activation of heat shock proteins. Heat shock proteins send an alarm call for the immune system to react to viral or bacterial invaders.

Even though the function of heat shock proteins is only partially understood, preliminary research suggest they help the body with both bacterial and viral infections, heart disease, neurodegenerative diseases like Alzheimer's, cancer and possibly many more diseases.

So it's clear that heat can play a key role in helping you fight off illness.

Now, you can try occasionally turning up your thermostat to 90 degrees… but if your spouse is anything like mine, you might be in for a pretty serious argument.

Your best bet is to do what I do — heat yourself with a near infrared sauna. This is the safest and best way to elevate your core body temperature for a therapeutic effect.

Not only is it possible to get the health benefits I just talked about, but sweating in a sauna is a superb detoxifier that removes metals, toxic chemicals, drugs, radioactive particles and other toxins out of the body.

For this reason alone I try not to go even one day without a sauna in our toxic world.

If you belong to a gym that has an infrared sauna, that's a great place to start.

Also, the prices on saunas have come way down over the past several years. Just Google "infrared sauna" and you'll find numerous opportunities to buy 1–2-person units for around $1,000.

Some units don't take up much more space than a large piece of furniture.

Maybe my taste buds aren't refined enough… or maybe I'm

LIKE TO BURN THAT STEAK? BETTER THINK AGAIN...

not as macho as some guys.

But I've never understood the desire to practically char meat until it looks like something you pulled out of a barn fire.

Who wants to taste a mouthful of ash — even if it's covered in barbecue sauce?

But if you're someone who likes to cook things "well done," it may be time to reconsider. Because science now proves that...

You may be literally cooking yourself to death!

Medical research shows that one way to dramatically reduce your risk of developing cancer is to avoid the tendency to consume overcooked foods.

We want everything fast in our culture, so cooking at high heat is very popular. But overcooking food actually produces cancer-causing compounds — and spending years eating this stuff puts your health at risk.

A group at the University of Minnesota reported that women who ate overcooked hamburgers had 50 percent greater risk of breast cancer than women who ate rare or medium-cooked hamburgers.

And the famous Iowa women's health study found that women who consistently ate well-done steak, hamburgers and bacon increased their risk of breast cancer nearly five-fold!

You men out there are also at risk. A study published in 2012 found that men who ate 1.5 servings of pan-fried meat each week increased their risk of advanced prostate cancer by 30 percent.

Men who ate 2.5 servings of red meat cooked at high temperature were 40 percent more likely to have advanced prostate cancer.

Considering that some of you guys out there are eating high-temperature, charred meat every single day may give us a clue about why prostate cancer rates are skyrocketing.

You see, cooking meats at high temperatures creates heterocyclic amines and these chemicals cause the mutation of genes. Heterocyclic amines have been linked to prostate, breast, colorectal, esophageal, lung and other types of cancer.

And it is important to remember that this doesn't just happen with red meat. If you grill salmon, which most of us consider a healthy food, you'll still get a big dose of heterocyclic amines.

Fortunately, there is a way to neutralize dietary carcinogens. One of the most potent chemicals is indole 3 carbinol (I3C) which is found in cruciferous vegetables like cabbage, cauliflower, brussels sprouts and broccoli.

Studies show that when you give I3C to rats before they are given cancer-causing chemicals, the number of tumors can be reduced by 96 percent.

So loading up on veggies at the family barbecue is probably a good idea. You can also buy I3C supplements on websites like **www.pipingrock.com.**

You'd be hard-pressed to find a bigger fan of pomegranates

SUPER FRUIT FIGHTS BREAST AND PROSTATE CANCER

than me.

I like pomegranates so much that I have five trees in my yard.

Of course, I love the taste — you get that hint of sweet and sour at the same time. But there's another reason I keep lots of pomegranates close by.

Pomegranates are a super fruit that can fight cancer, diabetes, heart disease, and MORE!

Scientists have discovered that pomegranates have various phytonutrients that have amazing health benefits.

One is ellagitannin, which inhibits the pro-inflammatory nuclear factor Kappa beta (NF-Kb). If NF-Kb is chronically elevated, it leads to inflammatory based diseases like cancer and diabetes.

But this isn't the only way that pomegranates can help keep you cancer-free.

Studies showed that pomegranates contain ellagic acid which functions to disrupt cancer development.

The seeds inhibit the aromatase enzyme which can

reduce your risk of breast cancer. Pomegranates also stimulate apoptosis of various cancer cells, which is where the cancer cell commits suicide.

A study was done where men with prostate cancer were given pomegranate juice to drink in one group and no pomegranate juice in the other group. They studied the time to doubling of the PSA level which tells how fast the cancer is growing.

In the control group without pomegranate juice it took 15 months for the PSA to double. In the group getting pomegranate juice it took 54 months for the PSA to double. **Pomegranate slowed the cancer development by more than 3 YEARS!**

Are urologists using this information in the treatment of prostate cancer? If they are, I haven't seen it in my patients.

Better still, pomegranates are great for your heart. Components in pomegranate juice increase PON-1, which helps with the function of HDL cholesterol which is the good cholesterol that cleans out our arteries.

Compounds in pomegranate also prevent oxidative damage to LDL-cholesterol which protects against atherosclerosis. Another way pomegranate can improve our blood vessels is by affecting the gene expression of nitric oxide synthetase. This results in increased nitric oxide which reduces the risk of developing plaque and leaves the arteries more flexible.

And lastly there's nutrition. Pomegranates are good source of vitamin C, potassium, B6 and pantothenic acid.

Pomegranates are powerful, natural disease fighters. And if you can't grow trees in your yard like I do, make sure you add pomegranates to your weekly grocery list.

Not too long ago, the American Cancer Society recommended

THE BREAST CANCER TEST YOU CAN SKIP (AND THE ONE YOU SHOULDN'T)

that women start getting mammograms at the age of 45 instead of 40.

And they nearly got their heads bitten off for it!

The breast cancer lobby is so powerful in America that speaking out against mammograms will get you labeled a quack in a hurry.

But they can call me what they want. Because there are some ugly truths about mammograms that millions of women aren't being told.

Chances are, you don't need a mammogram at all... maybe EVER!

I'll tell you all about a better alternative to mammograms in a moment. But first...

I have always thought that using mammograms — which expose the breast to ionizing radiation (a known cancer-causing agent) — is stupid.

The trouble with exposing the breast to radiation in younger women is that they will get more cumulative radiation, and therefore be more likely to reach the threshold forcausing cancer.

In addition, younger women tend to have denser breast tissue and therefore have more false-positive results which leads to worry and unnecessary, invasive procedures.

A 2012 study estimated that 70,000 women a year are plagued by false-positive tests.

And what about all those claims that mammograms are saving lives?

Well, the evidence is shaky at best.

There was a study reported in 2014 in the *British Medical Journal* that looked at 45,000 women between the ages of 40 to 59.

They compared using mammograms versus the usual care, which was having a yearly physical with your physician and no mammograms.

So what happened after 25 years? No difference in outcomes. In other words mammograms are completely ineffective at saving lives from breast cancer compared to just seeing your doctor and getting a physical.

I can see why the obstetrician and gynecologist groups want more mammograms. It's a way to get women engaged with the medical system, which is their bread and butter.

And why do groups like the Susan G. Komen Foundation want more mammograms done? Breast cancer is their business. They want to cure it. You can't cure what you haven't diagnosed.

They will give you statistics on how many lives are saved with heavy screening and early medical treatment.

But there is a hole in this argument. It has been shown that many of the breast cancers that are treated never would have killed the person.

This means a woman went through damaging treatment just because of the screening. When you enter these people into the data, they tend to survive so they boost the survival statistics.

But what is not seen in the studies, that I see every day in my practice, is all the damage that unnecessary treatment can do. There is chemo brain, depression, multiple health problems and a shorter life.

In my practice in Tucson, our first line of defense against breast cancer is a technology called digital thermography.

Most people have never heard of it, but this tool has been around for 35 years, more than 800 studies have been done on it, and Europe, Canada and Australia all use it for routine screening.

Thermography works by measuring infrared heat from your body and can be used over time to detect changes that occur.

One of its key benefits is that it detects cancerous changes in the body FAR EARLIER than a mammogram can — which gives you the best chance for recovery.

Unlike mammograms, digital thermography uses NO radiation and NO compression. And, unlike mammograms, thermography is 90 percent accurate.

And best of all, unlike mammograms, thermography (when added to regular breast health checkups) increases survival rate by 61 percent.

It costs less, too.

It's important to note that digital thermography can't diagnose cancer, but what it can do is safely tell you if something suspicious is going on.

Then — and only then — do I recommend getting a mammogram.

Before you expose your sensitive breast tissue to massive amounts of radiation, excessive pressure, unnecessary biopsies, and radical surgical procedures, talk to your doctor about thermography.

Finally, remember that one of the easiest ways to lower

your cancer risk is by decreasing your exposure to artificial light, like blue light.

This is the kind of light we get from TV screens, computers, tablets, smart phones, and modern light bulbs. Research has shown that this light, especially when you're exposed to it at night, creates melatonin shortages and other hormone changes that can lead to cancer.

That's why night-shift workers have such higher cancer rates.

Keeping these devices out of your bedroom at night, applying blue light filters (you can find them on any app store), and wearing blue light-blocking glasses at night are great ways to limit your exposure and possibly keep cancer from taking root.

CHAPTER FOUR

MAKE PAIN VANISH WITH THESE AMAZING TRICKS

SOOTHE ACHING JOINTS AND MUSCLES WITH THIS OLYMPIC ATHLETES' SECRET

I've spent my entire career treating pain — and researching new and better ways to do it.

I've helped marathon runners... elite Division I athletes at the University of Arizona... and countless seniors like you looking for relief from sore muscles and joints.

And for handling these thousands and thousands of pain cases, I had the best preparation you could imagine — I raised three active boys.

My sons played sports year-round, and they were always coming home with bruises, muscle pulls, strains, and other injuries.

And while treating my own sons I came across what may be the greatest pain breakthrough of my career.

It's called low-level light therapy, or LLLT. It's so effective at soothing even the worst pain that Olympic athletes rely on it to recover from injuries.

And if pain is controlling your life... and keeping you from enjoying the activities you love... LLLT may be the answer to your prayers.

Pain Sufferers See the Light

More than a decade ago — when my sons were tearing it up on the basketball courts and baseball diamonds — I had an incredible tool that most doctors didn't.

I'd been given a demonstration device that consisted of a panel of LED lights with a frequency of 630 nm. It was one of the early at-home LLLT devices.

And I quickly learned that LLLT had the power to…

Make pain and injuries vanish — almost like they'd never happened at all!

Whenever there was an injury (and there were many), we would strap on the LED panel and let it perform its magic.

My kids were often better the very next day and rarely missed practices or games.

And I wasn't the only doctor catching on to the amazing pain-relief properties of LLLT. I read recently that LED lights were regularly being used to quickly heal athletes at the Rio de Janeiro Olympic Games.

I guess my boys and I were ahead of our time!

Now, you may have heard that some physicians use another type of light treatment, called low-level laser therapy.

These treatments require going to a medical facility and are expensive.

These powerful devices have to be used with a lot of caution, because they can damage tissue, so you need an experienced provider.

Instead, I use LED lights with my patients, which are much safer and cheaper, while still providing the same benefits.

And the results have been remarkable. I've been relying on LLLT with LED lights for years, and I've seen this amazing treatment deliver fast results for muscle aches, arthritis, back problems, and just about every pain you can imagine.

The secret is that this light penetrates deep into your tissue to attack pain at the source.

Healing Pain 10 Different Ways

If you're skeptical about LLLT, I don't blame you. It doesn't seem like a simple panel of lights should be able to deliver such fast and complete pain relief.

And that's especially true if you've spent years trying just about every drug or therapy under the sun to treat your pain.

But the fact is, LLLT helps produce at least 10 amazing changes in your body that can help erase pain. Research has shown that LLLT...

1. Stimulates cytochrome C oxidase, an enzyme that releases ATP (the energy currency of our cells) and facilitates healing.
2. Helps our cells use energy better by creating an electrical charge in the water of our cells (we have Dr. Gerald Pollock at Washington State University to thank for this discovery).
3. Increases blood circulation.
4. Improves the transfer of vital nutrients to cells and damaged tissues.
5. Boosts the elimination of wastes and damaging free radicals.
6. Enhances the synthesis of collagen, an important building block for bones, muscles, and connective tissue.
7. Causes a tightening of the elastin and pores of the skin.
8. Activates stem cells, which are vital to repairing and replacing tissue.
9. Decreases scarring.
10. Lessens abnormal skin pigmentation.

So how does it all work? Well, this is where things get a little scientific — but stay with me.

You've heard before that light comes in lots of different frequencies or wavelengths.

The color of light is actually determined by the wavelength of the photons. The visual range wavelengths go from 380 to 700 nm.

Research has shown different benefits of the various wavelengths. Two beneficial wavelengths are the red light from 630 to 660 nm and the near-infrared frequencies from 810 to 830 nm which are just outside the visual spectrum.

The LLLT devices you'll see at doctors' offices or in at-home products will typically produce light at these wavelengths. As I shared with you, the earliest device I began using produced LED red light at 630 nm.

Both the red light and near-infrared frequencies are absorbed by the enzyme cytochrome C oxidase, triggering the healing mechanisms I discussed.

In other words, all light is not the same. To promote real healing, you need to have the correct wavelenth.

Buying the Right LLLT Device

There are some doctors out there like me who regularly use LLLT in our practices. But the treatment is so safe, that there are now plenty of at-home devices available.

You may be asking, "Dr. G, which device should I get?"

Unfortunately, there has been such an explosion of devices on the market that this question gets tougher and tougher to answer. It's nearly impossible to keep track of (and thoroughly review) them all.

But there are a couple of guiding principles you can follow.

There seems to be more benefit when the therapy is pulsed. LED red and infrared devices can be pulsed at frequencies of 10 Hz and 40 Hz, with both frequencies showing benefits.

There are also LED panels that emit the red and-near infrared frequencies mentioned above, like the one I used for my kids, which are good for strapping on to areas of injury or pain.

The Joovv high-powered, whole-body device is a great piece of at-home equipment for treating a variety of injuries (learn more at **www.joovv.com**).

An inexpensive way to use light therapy is to build your own near-infrared sauna with a 250-watt heat lamp that is available at home improvement stores.

In my home, I have a canvas sauna with a panel that has four of these 250-watt bulbs that I use for light therapy and sauna detox. You can pick one up at **www.saunaspace.com.**

These heat lamp bulbs contain light in the yellow, orange and red visible range, as well as invisible near-infrared and mid-infrared wavelengths.

As a rule of thumb, be sure to discuss any proposed therapy for a medical condition with your healthcare provider before using a light therapy device.

Bonus Content! The Versatility of Light Therapy

I predict that we will one day see LLLT as one of the greatest health breakthroughs of our time.

Not only does it improve tissue healing from injuries, it has been shown to have other uses including relief for:

- Muscle trigger points;
- Fibromyalgia pain;
- Inflammatory arthritis pain;
- Alzheimer's disease;
- Parkinson's disease;

- Skin tightening and wrinkle removal;
- Autoimmune thyroiditis (Hashimoto's disease);
- Hair loss;
- Macular degeneration;
- Kidney failure; and
- Peripheral neuropathy.

There are also devices that can improve overall health by irradiating the blood. The VieLight is inserted into the nostril to provide light therapy to the blood for general health. The treatment is generally 10 to 20 minutes per day.

You can learn more at **www.vielight.com.**

DON'T REPLACE THOSE PAINFUL JOINTS — START REBUILDING THEM!

Maybe your shoulder is so sore that even having a catch with your grandkids — or pulling weeds in the garden — is next to impossible.

Or those painful knees make even climbing a simple flight of stairs feel like torture.

And what does the mainstream medical establishment expect you to do?

They want to cover up the symptoms by putting you on dangerous and addictive painkillers... or they want to wheel you in for a joint replacement (followed by months of physical therapy).

Neither of these treatments are going to do a darned thing to address why your painful joints were failing in the worst place.

And in the case of surgery, you might come out of the operation in more pain and in worse shape than before! But what if you could...

Start repairing your painful joints in as little as *90 days flat!*

It's all possible, thanks to the work of Dr. Alan Moore.

Working in his own kitchen, trying to help a daughter who had rheumatoid arthritis, Moore developed one of the great joint breakthroughs of our time.

It's called UC-II, which is short for undenatured type II collagen (we call it CLG9), and it's actually derived from chickens.

That all may sound a little strange, but let me explain.

We know that collagen is an essential building block for the cushioning of our joints — but, like everything else, it can wear out over time.

The next thing you know, you have bone on bone — and even the smallest movements can leave you in agony.

Well, that's where UC-II comes to the rescue.

It delivers collagen straight to your joints, helping to rebuild the cushioning that can keep you pain-free and allow you to enjoy the active life you want.

And UC-II is blowing away other joint supplements on the market today!

In one study on patients with knee arthritis, published in the *International Journal of Medical Science*, patients experienced an unbelievable 40 percent improvement on a common measure of arthritis symptoms in just 90 days.

In fact, UC-II performed 2–3 times better than a combo of glucosamine and chondroitin (which are the leading joint supplements sold today).

What would it mean to you to know that smoother, more comfortable joints were just 90 days away? How long have you been popping those pain pills anyway?

Trust me, you'll never hear about UC-II from your typical mainstream doctor. But you can pick it up online or through your local vitamin and supplement shop.

You can buy NOW Foods UC-II at **www.puritan.com.**

NEVER GET KNEE SURGERY UNTIL YOU READ THIS

I know a thing or two about pain.

I've been lucky enough to climb some of the tallest peaks in the world — including in Alaska and the Himalayas — and you can't make it to the top without pushing through the pain.

But that kind of pain is temporary. I know that there are millions of Americans walking around with the kind of chronic pain that can wreck your quality of life on a daily basis.

And for those with chronic knee pain, climbing the stairs to the bedroom can seem as daunting as climbing the Himalayas.

So when doctors dangle the idea of knee replacement surgery, I can hardly blame someone for getting in line.

There's just one problem: It doesn't work.

And you could be headed for a major disappointment.

In a study published in *BMJ,* researchers studied approximately 4,500 patients between 45 and 79 who had knee replacements due to arthritis.

The overall consensus was that the surgery had only

minimal effects on quality of life — especially for those with less severe pain and loss of function.

That's a lot of pain... a lot of rehab... and a whole lot of dollars spent... for only "minimal effects."

This "discovery" has left some people in the medical community wondering if knee replacement is overused.

Overused? You must be kidding me!

Between 2000 and 2010, there was an 86 percent increase among men and a 100 percent increase among women. With more than 640,000 knees replaced per year, knee replacement surgery has become the most common inpatient procedure performed on people over 45.

That's the very DEFINITION of overused!

But I've got a better idea: Forget replacing your knee — fix it!

Obviously, a great place to start is with the low-level light therapy I discussed earlier in this chapter or UC-II. LLLT is fantastic at decreasing inflammation and stimulating your body's healing response.

Another treatment that works wonders — and that I regularly use in my practice — is called prolotherapy.

Prolotherapy is a simple procedure that basically injects sugar water into your painful joint. That actually directs your body's immune system to the area, where it can begin to repair some of the damage that's leaving you in pain.

I'll explain more about prolotherapy on page 97.

But here's what it's most important to know — prolotherapy directly impacts the underlying condition that's causing the pain in the first place. Unlike other treatments, which offer only short-term relief, prolotherapy offers long-term — and in some cases permanent — pain relief.

And while I've seen dramatic results in patients with knee pain, prolotherapy can be used to treat degenerative disorders in ANY of your joints, plus it can help with tendon issues, muscle strain, ligament sprains, meniscus tears, and even osteoarthritis!

Hands down, in my 35 years of medical practice, I've never seen a treatment for pain work as fast — or as well — as prolotherapy. Extensions of this are platelet rich plasma and stem cell injections. To find a provider you might try the website **getprolo.com**

Flip to page 97, and I'll tell you more about another exciting pain treatment and where you can get it.

THE "SUGAR WATER" SOLUTION FOR ERASING PAIN

In the previous article, I told you a little about prolotherapy — and how it may be a serious alternative for people considering knee surgeries or replacements.

And, trust me, I know what I'm talking about.

I can't tell you the number of patients I've treated who came to me only after they had a knee surgery fail.

Now, I'm going to share a little more about prolotherapy, variations of it, why it works, and where to get it.

But first, it helps to understand what's often causing your joint pain in the first place.

You see, research has shown that chronic pain is often caused by neuropathic pain.

What that means is that the nerves themselves are generating the pain signals and the nerves trigger inflammation around the surrounding tissues.

It may be your joints or muscles that hurt — but your nerves are the problem.

And this is a HUGE problem with knee and other joint replacements.

I often get patients that have had a total knee replacement for chronic pain.

Their knee STILL hurts after the operation and months of rehab. But their orthopedic doctor tells them that their artificial joint is fine and there's nothing they can do for the pain.

So they're placed on drugs or just have to tough it out. That's TOTALLY unacceptable for someone who just plunked down $35,000 for what was supposed to be a life-changing surgery.

But with careful examination, I usually find that the nerves that course over the surface of the muscles are swollen and tender. Again, it's not the joint that's the problem — it's the nerves.

Dr. John Lyftogt of New Zealand discovered that injecting dextrose (a type of sugar) solution over these painful nerves quickly relieves the pain and also diminishes the swelling of the nerve. This procedure was called neural prolotherapy (now he calls it perineural injections), and it stimulates your natural healing response in the nerve.

A series of these injections done weekly can *completely eliminate* the pain over a course of 5 or 6 weeks. That's right...

You can be pain-free in just 5–6 weeks!

I went through Dr. Lyftogt's training and have used perineural injection to relieve all sorts of pain for countless patients.

In addition to treating knees, I have saved many people from having to have surgery or powerful drugs for conditions like:

- Morton's neuroma (a common foot problem);
- Carpal tunnel syndrome;
- TMJ pain of the jaw;
- Shoulder pain;
- Migraine headaches; and
- Pain around the spine.

Because this treatment is so effective, I was performing this procedure six or more times a day just from patients that come in from word-of-mouth recommendations from other patients.

More recently Dr. Lyftogt discovered that mannitol (a type of sugar alcohol) injected over the nerves has some advantages over dextrose, and mannitol is what I now use in my practice.

Mannitol is very safe and is not metabolized in the body, so it doesn't affect blood sugar or diabetes.

In the thousands of injections that I've done, there's never been a side effect or bad reaction. This is one of the safest procedures a doctor can do.

Among the 600 or so doctors worldwide that perform these injections, the only adverse reaction has been a skin or subcutaneous infection estimated to occur in one out of every 300,000 injections.

In other words, I'll put the perineural injection safety record up against surgery or prescription drugs any day of the week.

Now can you imagine if all physicians knew about this simple, safe treatment that can be a life-changer for those with chronic pain? Yet this procedure is unknown by most pain specialists and nearly all general practitioners.

Find a specialist that has been trained by Dr. Lyftogt.

A great place to start is with the search tool at **http://www.lyftogtmed.com/where-to-get-lyftogt-pit/**

This treatment does not cure every type of pain, but it often cures chronic neuropathic pain which is one of the leading causes of chronic pain overall.

A good physician will perform a history and physical examination which will determine if you're a candidate for this therapy.

And you won't have to worry about wasting your time

with weeks of injections. We usually know after the first injections whether or not this is the right treatment for your pain.

And what if you're scared of needles? There are times when this treatment can be effective topically. What seems to be effective is a topical cream or gel with added mannitol and vitamin D3.

If you have a phobia of needles, talk this over with your doctor.

DON'T LET THIS QUICK PAIN FIX PUT YOUR LIFE AT RISK

It's become as big an American tradition as baseball or apple pie.

Just about everyone you meet is keeping a bottle of ibuprofen in their medicine cabinets or purses. We whip out these pills for everything from headaches to arthritis to simple exercise pain.

And it's all because we've been told that ibuprofen and other NSAIDs (nonsteroidal anti-inflammatory drugs) are safe.

After all, they wouldn't be sold over-the-counter if they were dangerous, right?

But what if EVERYTHING we've been told about OTC pain pills is a lie?

Not too long ago, even the Food and Drug Administration strengthened its warnings about the side effects of NSAIDs. This warning affects drugs you may be taking every day, like ibuprofen, naproxen, diclofenac, celecoxib and others.

These meds aren't nearly as safe as they're made out to be. And, in many cases, they're killers.

It is estimated that NSAIDs cause **16,000 deaths a year**

in the United States — mainly through gastrointestinal bleeding.

When you're taking an NSAID, you actually TRIPLE your chances of a potentially life-threatening gastrointestinal bleed.

And the risks don't stop there.

The new FDA warnings are now targeting how NSAIDs could make you a sitting duck for a heart attack or stroke.

Studies show the risk of a heart attack or stroke increases from 20 percent to 50 percent while you're taking these drugs, and the side effect can occur very early on.

About 30 billion doses of NSAIDs are taken a year are taken by Americans. So countless people are being put at risk.

Even worse, these drugs don't always work that well.

One of the big uses for NSAIDs is for treatment of arthritis pain. But there is some data that suggests that taking these drugs slows cartilage healing.

So, in essence, NSAIDs hasten the loss of cartilage that makes your joint problems worse.

Now I haven't lost my mind... at least not any more than usual. I don't expect you to just live with pain.

But there are plenty of other options for quick pain relief, including treatments and supplements you can try at home that are just as convenient.

A good standby is ice which is very effective at reducing pain and inflammation.

Krill oil supplements and niacinamide have been shown in studies to be about as effective as NSAIDs for treatment of arthritis pain (but a whole lot safer). You can pick them both up at **www.iherb.com.**

Also, don't forget this time-tested remedy from Doctor Mom — soak in Epsom salts. A good Epsom salt bath can raise your magnesium levels, and magnesium is one of the best solutions around for relaxing away muscle pain.

And for one of the best, natural inflammation-fighters around, just flip to my next article.

ELIMINATE INFLAMMATION WITH THIS DELICIOUS INDIAN SECRET

It's the kind of thing that should have Big Pharma executives drooling on their mahogany board room tables.

Imagine a wonder pill that could stop inflammation right at the source.

I'm talking about an easy and safe solution that could help tackle inflammatory diseases like arthritis… cancer… Alzheimer's disease… depression… and so much more.

One that's been proven in more than 600 rigorous scientific studies.

Well, this amazing cure already exists. But it was invented by our Creator, not a bunch of drug company lab technicians.

It's the Indian spice turmeric. And its active component curcumin is possibly the greatest inflammation-fighter on Earth.

Research has shown that curcumin and other turmeric extracts relieve pain and depression as well as prescription drugs, and absolutely destroy cancer cells in lab studies.

Now, as you probably know, turmeric is one of the main ingredients in curry.

And most Americans haven't grown up eating this spice like they do on the Indian subcontinent and in Asia.

After traveling to India, I developed a taste for it and so my kids got exposed to turmeric early. And adding turmeric to your diet is one of the smartest and healthiest things you can do.

But turmeric comes with a BIG problem — and most people don't know about it.

Turmeric is an absolute super-spice, but many of the main ingredients like curcumin are poorly absorbed from the gastro-intestinal tract. But this problem is easy enough to fix.

Studies have shown that your absorption of turmeric and curcumin are greatly improved (as much as seven-fold) if you combine them with black pepper, which has an active component called piperine. So black pepper can be added to either the spice or supplements.

I generally recommend trying to get the health benefits from turmeric by using the spice rather than the supplements, where you'll benefit from all the other compounds in the plant.

But if you have a medical condition that needs reversing like osteoarthritis, depression or other inflammation, you might consider purchasing a supplement that has curcumin with piperine or other modifications to make curcumin bioavailable.

1MD makes a formulation called Turmeric Curcumin Platinum, with a black pepper extract called BioPerine. You can find it at www.1md.org.

If you're not sure whether inflammation is a problem for you, a simple test can help. With my patients I test for highly sensitive C-reactive protein, as a guide to whether inflammation is a problem

My cut off for a healthy CRP is less than one.

CHAPTER FIVE

HEAL YOUR GUT, SHED POUNDS & LOOK GREAT!

DR. G'S 4-STEP WEIGHT-LOSS BOOT CAMP

If you've been struggling to shed some unwanted pounds… if you're tired of looking at that bulging belly or love handles… you know how hard it is to find reliable advice.

Everywhere we turn, we're surrounded by fad diets, magic pills, and workout contraptions that are supposed to melt away fat. And you've probably learned the hard way that most of what's out there today is junk… and some of it is a scam.

But your frustrating search for a permanent weight-loss solution ends today. Because I'm about to introduce you to…

A 4-step plan for WINNING the battle of the bulge!

This is a proven protocol I've used to help my own patients drop weight quickly and effectively — and they've dramatically improved their health as a result.

And it all starts with a hormonal problem that you probably never realized you had…

Step #1: Rebooting Your Leptin Sensitivity

Leptin is a critical hormone that is associated with obesity — and it's supposed to tell you when you're full.

But over time our cells can become resistant to leptin... they basically ignore it. When this happens, you are suffering from leptin resistance (LR).

The easiest way to determine LR is to look in the mirror. If you're overweight, you're LR.

If you still have a large appetite and crave carbohydrates, especially at night, you are also likely LR.

The good news is that you can reboot your leptin sensitivity, which is the first step in losing weight.

To regain leptin sensitivity, follow a low-carbohydrate diet and strictly limit grains. By doing this, you're eliminating the foods that cause leptin receptors to become nonfunctional.

Have breakfast within 30 minutes of waking. Make sure it is low in carbs (less than 50 grams), has a lot of protein, and it can have fat. I recommend a minimum 50 grams of protein for most people.

You can tell how much is right for you by looking at your hunger later in the day. If you remain hungry throughout the day, you need to eat more protein in the morning.

If you can skip lunch and dinner, you're probably overdoing protein at breakfast.

As for protein sources, pastured or organic eggs are good and/or grass fed meats, poultry, offal or fish. A third option, although less ideal, would be whey protein or other protein shakes, minus the fruit or sugar.

Try to limit total carb intake to 25 grams if you are overweight by more than 30 lbs.

If you are fit and have a small amount of weight to lose, (less than 30 lbs.) you can increase your carb loads. Most people will be able to eat carbs eventually, but try to avoid starches and sugar until you have mastered your cravings and hunger.

And here's the best part — you don't need to count calories.

Any time you eat carbs, use liberal amounts of ghee, butter, heavy cream, coconut or palm oil. Coconut oil is good because of the metabolism-boosting effects of medium chain triglycerides, and it helps heal the gut.

How and when you eat your fuel is more important than any other factor, including the food itself.

Eat 3 meals per day and avoid snacking. It takes insulin about 3 hours to go down, so that the body can begin to burn fat. So you need to have 4 to 5 hours between meals so that your body learns to go into the fat-burning mode. Spacing meals gives the pancreas time to build up insulin for the next meal.

Eating snacks causes the release of insulin and stresses the pancreas.

Some people will be too unhealthy to start with 3 meals a day, because of low blood sugar levels. If this is you, start with 4 meals a day and then, as you improve, move to 3.

Try to allow 3–5 hours between the evening meal and sleep time. If you eat too late, or too much, you will disrupt autophagy (cell repair) that occurs during sleep. Without autophagy optimized, you will age faster and eventually start to gain weight and develop modern diseases.

Most people will notice a change in their cravings and hunger within 4–8 weeks.

So how will you know that you're becoming leptin sensitive again?

You will notice positive mood changes first and then sleep will improve. Clothes will fit differently but weight may not change drastically initially. Weight loss will generally come if you continue the program.

You will have better recovery from exercise and your energy levels will improve.

When you awaken you will feel refreshed like you slept well.

When these signs are all present you can begin or add more exercise.

In the beginning, you may have to force yourself to follow the rules. As time goes on and your cravings decrease, it becomes much easier.

Step #2: Cold Adaptation Protocol

My cold adaptation protocol can be used for an aide to weight loss. This is an extension of the leptin reboot that I just described.

Not everyone needs cold adaptation, but I believe it can be beneficial for virtually everyone. I have been doing this myself for years.

Skin cooling sends a message to the brain which induces fat cell death and subsequent loss of subcutaneous fat without damaging the overlying skin or the underlying muscle layers. Cold also causes rapid leptin sensitivity.

With cold stimulus, fat is forced to liberate leptin from fat cells. This is new scientific information that was first studied in pigs in 2008, and subsequently tested in humans and found to be quite effective for fat removal in selected areas of the body.

Cold therapy (often called cold thermogenesis, or CT) forces the brain to slowly rewire in the hypothalamus to burn all excessive WAT (white adipose tissue), and induces the formation of BAT (brown adipose tissue). BAT contains mitochondria which burn fat to produce heat.

In other words, ***BAT is the good stuff that helps burn unwanted fat.***

Before you begin CT, you must make sure your cardiac risks are low and there are other risks to consider such as hypothermia, frostbite and drowning. Talk things over with your doctor and you may need a family member or friend as a spotter. Most people will be able to do this at home.

First, you must choose the right environment for your CT. Cold water is 24 times more effective than cold air.

I usually do my training in the late afternoon or after nightfall after dinner.

Phase 1: The easiest way to start CT is to first place your face in ice cold water as you monitor the time of exposure. You should not use makeup or facial products before face-dunking. You need thermometer, ice, a bathroom sink or large bowl, and a watch or timer.

Enter face first and see how long you can tolerate the cold water using a time piece. I repeat this several times for a total of about 5 minutes of face submersion. For the next two weeks work your way up until you are able to stay under for as long as you can hold your breath. You will notice your ability to hold your breath will improve with this training.

When the skin becomes pale, it may mean that your temperature is going too low. So watch your skin color. When it begins to get to pale, end the session then.

Phase 2: After you've spent some weeks mastering phase 1 you're ready for phase 2, place 10–20 lbs. of ice on your torso. This sensitizes you quickly to cold.

This might be hard at first. Try to extend your time by 5 minutes each session until you get to 60 minutes. You will notice your skin is pink to cherry red and numb in places.

If you develop cold urticaria (hives), this is a sign you have high levels of tissue and serum omega 6 fats or your body has lost energy from EMF/artificial light causing dehydration. Stop the experiment and adjust your technology exposure and alter your diet.

If you don't develop cold urticaria, proceed on to see how long you can tolerate the cold. Make sure you have no metal on your torso or ears or nose when you do this. Record your times, and pay attention to your skin color.

After ten minutes, you will notice numbness and tingling present on these cold areas. As your times increase, you may notice numbness in areas adjacent to the ice develop, too.

This usually occurs with longer exposures and with more surface area covered on your skin. The length of time you expose yourself should be matched to how much extra fat you have.

The more overweight you are, the longer your exposure should be. You want your skin to always remain pink to cherry red when you are doing this. If it gets pale you need to stop the test and take a warm shower.

When you can tolerate the skin being covered for one hour with pink to cherry red skin, you're now ready for the Cold Tub step.

Phase 3: Once you complete Phase 2, you can try cold showers or baths. I started by filling the bathtub with cold tap water.

At first I kept my hands and feet out of the tub. The head can represent a significant site of heat loss.

I then proceeded to add 20 pounds of ice to my chest and abdomen region while my body was in the tub. Initially, I kept my socks and gloves on my extremities, and I also wore a knitted cap on my head. This was all to combat the vasoconstriction that normally will occur in your extremities.

After I was adapted to 20 pounds of ice (about 7 days), then I removed socks, gloves, and head cap. If you get lightheaded, this means you're not ready for the tub. Abort the tub and go back to dunking your face in the cold water.

If you can handle the 20 pounds of ice, you can increase it by 10 pounds of ice at a time to cover more of your body with icy water. This process is trying to use the peripheral nervous system's cold receptors in the skin to tell the brain something has radically changed in the current environment.

After you can get past 20–45 minutes of this, you will notice your tolerance to cold dramatically changes in water, air, and in ice. You will be able to wear less clothing and go outside and not be cold.

At 45 minutes, you can choose to stop and then plan on doing this 2–5 times a week depending upon your starting weight, body fat, and what your goals are. Always expose the fat areas of your body to the cold water.

Another way to cold adapt is to cover the upper body with ice bags on the torso, while the bottom half is submerged in the water of a hot tub. You sit in warmer water while the upper half of the body is completely exposed to the elements (if it's cold) or otherwise packed with ice on the chest and abdomen. It is very effective at lowering your surface temperatures but you are not as cold overall.

You burn a lot more calories when it's cold outside, so you should get outside in cold and try not to bundle up with clothing as you adapt.

In the beginning of winter, most people wear a ton of clothing when they go outside in cold weather. Don't wear so much clothes and think of shivering as a good thing. The more leptin resistant one is, the more the cold will help.

The beauty of this adaptation is that is does not require any change to your core temperatures. When you begin to mess with your core temperatures, you can get into trouble with frostbite and freezing injury.

Step #3: Getting the RIGHT Kind of Exercise

Exercise is the part of weight loss that most people enjoy the least.

The good news about exercise is that most of the benefit occurs with mild to moderate amounts. The benefit curve flattens significantly when exercise is intense and prolonged.

In other words, really pushing hard does not give much added benefit.

In fact, studies show that recreational exercisers have their immune system stimulated so they tend to have fewer colds and flus. One study showed they got sick at only 50 percent of the rate of sedentary people.

The highly trained endurance athlete, however, has 4.5 times more colds and flus than the sedentary person. So the lesson here is...

More exercise is NOT necessarily better... or healthier.

Is exercise critical for weight loss? It can be helpful, but I have had people lose tons of weight without doing much in the way of exercise.

More than half of my weight-loss clients have adrenal burnout. For these people, vigorous exercise is not recommended. Adrenal burnout is best evaluated by a salivary Adrenal Stress Index test and other labs that I do, like sex hormones, salivary melatonin, IGF-1, C reactive protein, Free T3, Reverse T3, RBC magnesium and 25 OH vitamin D.

Many people that have adrenal burnout use exercise as one would use coffee or cigarettes for stimulation. It can be very hard to face the truth that they need to quit doing vigorous exercise and address their burnout instead. Addressing adrenal fatigue is important to re-balance the body so it will release excess fat.

For people with adrenal burnout and sympathetic dominance (the "fight or flight" nervous system in over-drive), I recommend only light exercise such as walking and a minimal amount of strength work.

This doesn't mean that you will never be able to do vigorous exercise again. Once your labs show that your body is more balanced and your energy producing mito-chondria and glands (thyroid and adrenals) are at opti-mal levels, you'll have a tremendous urge to exercise and that's when you can begin to do vigorous exercise.

Outdoors is the best place for exercise. Gyms can be good for strength exercises, stretching or exercise classes, but they have the disadvantage of more artificial light expo-sure which in most people is already at unhealthy levels.

One of the best ways to incorporate movement is to do it as part of your daily living activities. Walk more, take stairs and lift things. The obsession of putting everything on rollers is kind of ridiculous.

We pay money to go to a gym to do the same lifting we could have done at the grocery store.

The best time to exercise is the late afternoon, although this isn't usually the most convenient time. Early in the morning, when many people exercise, is not ideal because the collagen structure of our connective tissue is swollen and unstable.

This is because of normally elevated levels of cortisol in the early morning. Daily morning sun exposure helps to re-zip collagen so that it is stronger for exercise later in the day and it stays that way because people normally have low cortisol in the late afternoon.

For those who are healthy enough, I recommend ideally at least one day a week of vigorous, endurance activities such as hiking up a hill, swimming, a long bike ride or running or power-walking 3–4 miles.

At least one day a week should be strength training where you perform repetitions with resistance until muscle fatigue of the major muscle groups including the extremities and back.

This can be accomplished using free weights, machines or exercises that utilize your own body weight.

For the other days of the week, do an activity at a light to moderate intensity that you enjoy such as walking, jogging, sports, dance, hiking, gardening or household chores.

Swimming can be good but there may be toxin exposure from pools that are treated with chemicals. Swimming in lakes, rivers and the ocean is usually better.

To summarize, the most important aspects of exercise/ movement:

1. Try to do activities that are fun and that you enjoy;
2. Do endurance activities at least once a week;
3. Do strength activities at least once a week;
4. Be active every day, most of the day, and;
5. Promote the flexibility of your connective tissue contained in bones, joints, muscles, tendons and ligaments by doing a variety of movements that take your joints to the limits of range of motion, preferably daily.

Step #4: Meditation

Meditation exercises can be very helpful in reducing mental /emotional pain and disturbances, which recent research shows contribute to poor health and weight gain.

Studies of meditation show that it can reduce cortisol levels. Cortisol is the stress hormone and its overproduction can result in insomnia, increasing abdominal fat and a weakening of connective tissue.

There are various ways to meditate. A simple way is to sit in a chair with your back straight.

Close your eyes and focus on your breathing. Take a series of slow breaths, feeling your abdomen push out as you inhale and moving in with each exhalation. Empty your mind of any thoughts. When you do this you may become aware of thoughts or emotions.

Once you realize a thought or emotion has taken over your mind or body, gently pull yourself back to focusing on your breathing and try to sense the energy field within your body.

If it helps, in the beginning you might want to visualize breathing in light into your body.

Alternatively, you can visualize a sphere the size of a basketball bisecting your body at the waist. Place your hands on the ball as you clear out thoughts from your consciousness.

You'll feel a tingling in your hands as you do this.

Every time a thought or emotion pops into your consciousness, acknowledge what it is but don't judge it or analyze it. Just return your focus to your hands on the ball and your breathing and the energy field within your body.

If you practice this for 10 or 15 minutes once or twice a day, with time you will be able to go deeper and better feel your internal energy.

Remember, eventually you want to feel your internal energy field rather than visualize it. This simple exercise can greatly reduce stress in your life, and that facilitates emotional health and weight loss.

NEVER FALL FOR THIS WEIGHT-LOSS SCAM

Quick fixes never work. Not in life, not in relationships, and certainly not in medicine.

That's why I am 100 percent against gastric bypass surgery.

I've seen the results too many times, and they are never good. People end up broken, sick, and literally shells of themselves.

So when I read about a recent study presented by the American Heart Association, I got up in arms.

According to the research, weight loss surgery is tied to lower risk of heart failure. A study like this could push someone who's been on the "should-I-or-shouldn't-I" line right on over the edge — and that's exactly what I'm afraid of.

But don't be fooled by the flashy headline.

The study compared two groups of obese people: one got weight loss surgery, the other dieted. At the end of four years, the group who got the gastric bypass surgery had a lower risk of heart failure.

But here's what they didn't tell you... both groups had a similar rate of heart attack and death!

That's right — they want you to believe this surgery is saving lives, but there's no evidence of that at all.

And here's what else this study doesn't mention…

- Roughly 1 in 200 die from complications during the surgery.
- Up to 10 percent need a second surgery.
- Up to 40 percent have problems ranging from diarrhea to hernias to intestinal leaks.
- Many develop abdominal pain because of adhesions.
- And patients can develop nutrient deficiencies because the bypass shrinks the areas of the intestinal tract that absorb nutrients, forcing them to take vitamins for the rest of their lives.

But wait, there's more! Even with all the risks and complications, the surgery itself rarely helps people accomplish the very task they are trying to achieve: losing weight!

Fewer than 10 percent of the people who have this surgery ever reach a healthy, "normal" BMI. And a shocking number gain the weight back after the first year.

Now that's mainstream medicine at its finest!

People who become morbidly obese have more serious underlying issues that no quick-fix surgery is going to erase. Toxins, stress, nutrient-poor diet, lack of rest — and the big one, emotional problems — can't be surgically removed.

Obese people also face another major roadblock when it comes to weight loss — they are leptin resistant. Leptin is a hormone that sends a signal to your brain when you've had enough to eat. When you're leptin resistant, your levels are high, but your brain isn't listening to it.

In other words, the switch that tells you to stop eating is broken.

Weight loss surgery can't fix it — but I'll tell you what can.

There's a protocol that works to reset leptin sensitivity, and it's as simple as 1–2–3:

1. Have a high protein breakfast
2. Eat three meals a day, no snacking, and no eating in the evening.
3. Those meals should be low carb.

After just weeks of following this protocol, your leptin receptors will wake up, and those cravings will go away.

Of course, no weight loss program is a quick fix, but getting your body's hormones to work WITH you, rather than AGAINST you, is a big step in the right direction.

THE WAR ON STOMACH ACID COULD BE KILLING YOU

I swear, the way Big Pharma operates is like an episode of "Let's Make a Deal."

They're always asking you to trade one health problem for another.

Only, with this game, you might not even realize you're playing until it's too late.

Case in point? Those heartburn meds you see advertised on TV around the clock.

The **15 MILLION people** taking proton pump inhibitors or H2 blockers to treat heartburn and acid reflux are placing themselves at risk every single day.

These drugs represent some of the biggest names in OTC and prescription drugs — names like Prilosec, Nexium, and Zantac, to name a few. The fact that they've become household names makes most people assume they're safe.

The science says otherwise.

According to a study published in the *JAMA Internal Medicine* that included over 7,700 patients, 22 percent of patients taking acid-suppressing drugs had recurrent infections with *C. difficile,* a potentially deadly type of bacteria.

The lucky ones who are infected with *C. difficile* only experience mild diarrhea and cramping. The not-so-lucky are faced with severe diarrhea, fever, kidney failure, and life-threatening inflammation of the colon.

Once you've been infected with *C. difficile,* your chances of getting it again skyrocket.

And do you know who's most at-risk? You guessed it — older adults!

But increased risk of *C. difficile* infection only scratches the surface of the dangers of these drugs. They've also been linked to muscle weakness, nutrient deficiencies, and an increased risk of food poisoning — not to mention pneumonia and kidney disease.

I have just one word for those findings: DUH!

Stomach acid may be painted as the enemy, but that's a myth the pharmaceutical industry has been selling ever since they developed drugs that worked to suppress stomach acid. The truth is, your body NEEDS stomach acid to help digest food and to help protect against any pathogens that are ingested.

Reducing this important ally to good health is like taking away your stomach's defensive line and then wondering why your opponent keeps scoring touchdowns.

No mystery there. By reducing stomach acid, you're intentionally making yourself more vulnerable to nutritional deficiencies and infection — including infection with *C. difficile.*

"What's the big deal?" you might be wondering. "If I contract an infection, I can just take an antibiotic."

Not so fast.

The use of antibiotics has lulled people into a false sense of security where infections are concerned, and we're all about to be in for a rude awakening. Overuse and misuse of antibiotics have given rise to what have come to be called "antibiotic-resistant superbugs."

Not too long ago, a woman had an infection that was resistant to ALL 26 antibiotics available in the U.S. She died.

I'm sorry to say her case isn't unusual. More than 700,000 people die every year from drug-resistant infections.

With drug-resistant superbugs on the rise, we should be increasing our body's defenses against dangerous infections — yet with drugs like proton pump inhibitors, we're doing just the opposite.

Quitting PPIs is one of the best things you can do for your long-term health. But don't do it cold turkey, or you can make the problem worse — work with your doctor on a plan to taper off.

HERE'S THE REAL CULPRIT BEHIND ACID REFLUX

My patients are always a bit surprised when I drop this little bomb: Acid reflux is rarely caused by excess stomach acid.

That's right. The premise that multiple drug companies have used to sell BILLIONS of dollars' worth of drugs is a BIG. FAT. LIE.

To understand why, we have to understand the root cause of acid reflux.

Remember, stomach acid is your friend — but only when it stays in your stomach. If it leaves the boundaries of your stomach, it quickly turns into the enemy.

That's because while the lining of the stomach was built to withstand the harsh acid environment, your esophageal lining is much more delicate.

When acid travels from your stomach up into your esophagus, it can cause a sharp pain or burning sensation severe enough to resemble a heart attack.

But the problem isn't the acid itself; the problem is that the acid is in the wrong place.

There's a circular muscle called the lower esophageal

sphincter that joins your esophagus and stomach. When you're eating, this valve opens up in order to allow food to travel to the stomach. At all other times, it should be shut tight.

If that flap stays open, acid flows in the wrong direction, and that's where your problems begin.

When the lower esophageal sphincter remains open, it allows oxygen into the stomach and plays havoc with our gut flora, which is essential for good health.

Despite the pervasive myth about excess stomach acid causing acid reflux, the REAL problem is a loose sphincter.

So what causes a loose sphincter?

Glad you asked.

In many cases, *the answer is simple as a deficiency in the mineral magnesium.*

Magnesium deficiency is rampant in America, with some estimates indicating that 90 percent of Americans are deficient. I can verify from personal experience it is rare that a patient has adequate levels of this important mineral.

Because magnesium plays a role in over 300 biochemical reactions in the body, this deficiency represents a serious health problem that impacts some of the most critical aspects of our health, including cardiovascular health, metabolism, and immune function.

But how it relates to acid reflux has to do with its role in maintaining healthy muscles. A magnesium deficiency can cause some or all of your muscles to be too tight or to spasm — including your lower esophageal sphincter.

Making matters worse, proton pump inhibitors are known for causing magnesium deficiency, which means they're exacerbating one of the underlying causes of the condition.

It's a good idea to get your magnesium levels checked with the RBC magnesium test. And, if needed, consider supplementing with magnesium (magnesium threonate is a form that's highly bioavailable).

In most cases, you can fix acid reflux without popping a single PPI — and at a fraction of the cost. Here's how:

4 steps to treating heartburn without drugs:

1. Chew your food! The more you chew, the less work your stomach has to do. Sound too simple to be true? Try it for one week and you'll be shocked at the difference.

2. Drink less with meals. Hydrating during meals dilutes your stomach acid, making it less potent. As a result, undigested food can stick around and start fermenting, causing gas to build up and push the lower esophageal sphincter open.

3. Avoid problem foods. Some foods are more likely to contribute to acid reflux: spicy foods, citrus, coffee, soda, fried foods, and refined starches — in other words, many of the foods you should be avoiding anyway!

4. Supplement with magnesium. Magnesium deficiency is one of the root causes of acid reflux. Be sure to avoid magnesium oxide, a common ingredient in many magnesium supplements. Instead, get a chelated magnesium like magnesium glycinate in a dosage of 200–800 mg per day. You'll know if it is too much for your system if you get loose stools.

THE ONE "HEALTH FOOD" YOU SHOULD NEVER EAT (YOU'LL BE SURPRISED...)

When you're trying to lose weight — or just improve your health — you'll get lots of advice on foods that are supposedly good for you.

But there's one that I want you to avoid, and you'll probably be a little shocked.

I'm talking about apples.

Yep, I'm sure mom told you a million times that eating an apple a day could keep the doctor away. But the problem is, I'm just not sure that's true anymore.

Do you ever notice how when you cut up a nice fresh apple, sometimes even the best apples seem to turn brown after just a few minutes, even if you put them in the refrigerator?

Thanks to new technology, you will not have to suffer eating brown apples any longer. But you're inheriting lots of other problems in the bargain.

Scientists in Canada genetically modified the apple by introducing a gene that creates resistance to an antibiotic, kanamycin.

That happens to disable the enzyme that leads to the browning of apples.

They call it the Arctic Apple and its genetic modification will be perpetrated on several different varieties of apples.

The advantages are that sliced apple products will maintain the appearance of freshness much longer. This is good for food producers and grocery stores.

The inventors plan to use it in baby food (yeah, that's a good group to experiment on).

So what about the safety studies? Well, unfortunately, GMOs never need safety testing under the current law.

With no testing, it's possible these apples are poisonous to some degree... we'll never know until it's too late. Maybe after they've sold a million pounds of applesauce for babies.

It's possible that the gene responsible for the non-browning of apples will transfer to our gut bacteria as has been seen in other genetic modifications in food plants.

And since this gene is associated with antibiotic resistance, I could see where this could be another problem with more antibiotic resistant germs.

Also, these apples will likely cross-pollinate with other apples, including organic apples. With this scenario, the long-term outcome could be that GMO apples are the only apple in existence.

Apples are a fruit I generally recommended avoiding even before I ever heard of the Arctic Apple.

If you look at the Environmental Working Group's list of the "dirty dozen" fruits and vegetables, apples are always near the top of the list.

There are 42 different pesticides found on apples and they are sprayed frequently. They also can have high herbicide residues.

There used to be multiple varieties of wild apples (back when mom spoke so highly of them). Because of our interference with hybridization, many of the wild apple varieties have become extinct.

Hybridization has increased the sugar content of apples, but decreases their vigor and now they rely on chemicals for survival.

If you do have an apple, be sure that it's organic and tree ripened. And it is best to have a wild or heirloom variety for it to give the good nutrition for which it was designed.

My advice to you would be to boycott the GMO apple and all other GMO foods until independent, adequate studies have been completed. I must admit however, even if studies were completed, I still believe it is too risky to genetically modify our food plants and animals.

I feel there are much safer ways to improve our food supply using small-scale farms applying ecological, sustainable agricultural practices.

AVOID GUT PROBLEMS WITH THIS SIMPLE DRINKING TRICK

Here's a quick health tip that I use in my practice to help my patients keep their guts healthy and properly digest their food.

Do you ever notice that in restaurants, they bring you a big glass of ice water? And then, if you have good waiter, they keep it full no matter how many times you empty it.

We've always thought that drinking lots of water with our meals is helpful. But not so fast

Having freezing water paralyzes your stomach to some extent, so ice is a no-no if you want your stomach to function properly.

I recommend minimizing water up to 15 minutes before meals and for two hours after, so that you give your digestive tract the best chance to digest your food.

You've heard that we are what we eat… but, really, we are what we digest.

Minimizing water and other beverages with meals keeps us from diluting our stomach acid, digestive enzymes and bile salts.

Most people have their digestion substantially damaged by our nutrient-poor diet of processed foods and the disruption of our biochemistry through toxins.

I also recommend, if you have digestive problems, supplementing at meals with digestive enzymes.

Doctor's Best makes digestive enzymes that you can pick up at websites like **www.iherb.com.**

HERE'S ONE WEIGHT-LOSS GIMMICK YOU'LL WANT TO AVOID

If you're struggling to lose weight, constant hunger is your worst enemy.

I can't tell you how many patients I've treated who complain that they're hungry all the time... even shortly after meals.

Now, some doctors are offering a high-tech new way to control those hunger cravings.

And my advice? Run for the hills — FAST!

The method is called Maestro, and it's like having a cattle prod inserted in your chest that zaps your vagus nerve so you don't feel hungry. That's how you lose weight.

The medical system is desperate to find profitable ways to help us lose weight and that's because we're in the middle of an obesity epidemic.

Everyone wants to slow down the obesity problem, but no one seems to want to address the causes. They just want to find a treatment, no matter how expensive or risky it is.

If you look at the reports on Maestro, they talk about how there is a 25 percent EWL, which stands for extra weight loss.

Of course, that sounds impressive… but here's what they're not telling you. The placebo group lost weight, too, so the Maestro only accounted for about an extra 6 pounds of weight loss for a 200-pound person.

You're talking about spending thousands of dollars for every extra pound you lose. No thanks!

And how about the risks?

It's always risky to get sliced open, but especially when you're overweight.

Another factor is the electromagnetic field (EMF) exposure from the device. I'm constantly trying to get my patients to avoid EMFs, and the last thing I want them to do is to have their cell phone implanted under their skin.

That to me would risk cellular disruption from these electromagnetic fields.

Other risks that I could imagine are the adverse effects of having a key nerve in the body that is a critical part of our autonomic nervous system artificially stimulated over time and disrupting its normal function.

The 18-month study shows us almost a one-in-20 chance of a major adverse event, 4.3 percent to be exact.

I have a theory that is backed up by a lot of science, and also common sense, that the causes of obesity include circadian rhythm disruptions (including disruptions from EMFs), nutrient-poor diet, too much sugar and processed oils in the diet, toxins (now termed obesogens), stress and infections.

Yes, I know it's hard to address these causes… but having a cattle prod inserted into you is no picnic either.

THIS "MORNING MIRACLE" CAN HELP KEEP YOU TRIM

When I treat overweight patients, they're usually surprised by my first recommendation.

It doesn't involve scarfing down health foods or hiring some pricey personal trainer.

I tell them to get out in the sun… every single day.

You'll hear me talk about the benefits of sun exposure a lot, and there's a very good reason.

Adequate sun exposure can mean the difference between living to a ripe old age — or not.

The best hours appear to be in the morning, and this is particularly beneficial in the spring and summer.

I've talked before about the effects of the sun, which includes how it impacts hormones and the production of vitamin D.

And a study published in *PLOS One* gives us evidence of morning sun exposure's impact on body weight.

This is a study that was done on people who were fitted with a wrist device to monitor light exposure.

The bottom line of the study was that those people with

more morning sun exposure weighed significantly less than those that either did not get sun exposure or had their sun exposure in the afternoon.

So here we have a study backing up what I have been recommending and what I have found to help my patients with weight loss.

There is a caveat with sun exposure. Having adequate DHA in cell membranes is critical for making use of the energy from the sun.

This means you should be eating seafood on a regular basis if you want to be able to tolerate a full dose of sunlight, which optimally might be one or more hours per day.

At the same time of your sun exposure, I recommend that you be grounded to the Earth (this sounds a little "out there," I know, but hear me out).

Your body actually gets energy this way, and the more energy you have, the less your body has hoard by making blubber.

You ground by going barefoot on the dirt, grass, beach or on concrete. Asphalt is an insulator so it doesn't allow adequate grounding.

So here's a simple strategy that you can put in place today. Yes, you need to make it a priority, and somehow get it into your schedule, if you want to get the health benefits.

You can explore near-infrared lights and full-spectrum lighting if you absolutely can't get out in the sun.

WHY BACTERIA ARE A DIET'S BEST FRIEND

You've heard before about the trillions of healthy "gut bugs" or bacteria throughout your digestive system, and how important they are to immune function and properly digesting food.

But did you also know they could be the key to helping you lose those love handles for good?

There are many studies that show that obese people tend to have gut flora changes compared to lean people.

In fact, in one study researchers took the gut flora from an obese person and transplanted it into a mouse. And guess what? The mouse got fat.

Studies have shown that obese people often have lower bacterial species diversity in their gut. So it's important to understand a couple of factors that might alter species diversity and lead us down the path to obesity.

Obesity is closely related to type II diabetes. A recent case-control study showed that antibiotic use led to a 53 percent increase in diabetes.

It's obvious that antibiotic use can severely alter our gut

flora and can wipe out species that should be there.

Another study of over 1 million people reported in the *European Journal of Endocrinology* in 2015 showed a 37 percent increase in diabetes with increased antibiotic exposure.

I know I've been getting better in my medical practice about not giving antibiotics for every cold, sinus infection and ear infection. Especially when the trials that compare using antibiotic versus placebo for these conditions show no significant difference between taking antibiotics and not taking them.

And if you're a meat eater and don't eat organic meat, studies show you'll still get a healthy dose of antibiotics. You see, antibiotics are given to animals from factory farms, because it makes them fat, too, and they gain weight faster.

It's all about profits for these companies — this stuff is sold by the pound.

So if you eat animal meat from factory farms, you get the same antibiotics into your system, and evidence points to antibiotics being a major contributor to obesity and diabetes.

There's also a dietary practice that reduces the species diversity in our microflora. That's eating sugar, refined starch and fruit.

There is a molecule that's made in the liver, muscles and intestine that is increased when the food supply is low so that it stimulates the burning of fat.

This is called Fasting Induced Adipose Factor, or FIAF.

Studies show that when you eat a lot of refined starch and sugar, bacteria in the gut decrease their production of FIAF and you get fat. The fat cell produces more leptin as it gets bigger, which, in an ideal situation, should turn off our hunger.

But if there's any increased inflammation in the brain, which is very common, we develop leptin resistance and obesity. It would help here to eat a higher fat diet so that you starve the gut bacteria and they, in turn, produce more FIAF, which will cause us to burn fat and lose weight.

There's another factor involved in the gut flora that medicine has pretty much missed. There are many studies that show that UV light kills bacteria.

But what most people don't know, including doctors, is that the enterocyte cells that line our gut emit UV light. And studies show that the UV light given off by these cells is increased when you are in poor health, like when you have increased inflammation in your body.

So even if you don't take any antibiotics, you might still be at risk for having low gut bacterial diversity because you live in an inflammatory environment.

That means you have to get back to the ultimate cause of inflammation. Diet plays a role, but so does the crazy increase in electromagnetic field exposure in our high-tech life.

Studies show non-native electromagnetic fields (EMFs) cause inflammation even at low doses.

Another important factor in inflammation is circadian rhythm disturbances caused by artificial light at night.

There are short-term ways to increase your gut diversity, such as probiotics that are available from supplement companies.

There are foods with living, healthy organisms, such as yogurt, Kiefer, kimchi and sauerkraut.

Soil organisms also play a role. So if you have a garden, don't wash off the vegetables perfectly and then eat them raw to get some of those soil organisms. I don't recommend doing this with commercially grown produce.

Prebiotics feed your flora, and we commonly think of fiber. Fiber from asparagus, artichoke, garlic and root vegetables are particularly good.

Many of the grains, especially wheat, are inflammatory and their fiber should be avoided if you have gut problems.

CHAPTER SIX

HOW TO HAVE MIND-BLOWING SEX AFTER 60

THIS TESTOSTERONE LIE IS KILLING YOUR SEX LIFE

Remember those good, old days?

You were young, in shape, and ready for sex at a moment's notice.

But if you're like a lot of guys, somewhere along the way your "swinging 20s" turned into your "slumping 60s."

Lots of older guys who come into my office confess that they've practically lost interest in sex... and in the rare cases when they do have sex, they struggle to perform.

Their relationships and their self-esteem are suffering.

The good news is that there's a...

Safe, natural way to kickstart your sex life back into action!

But first you need to forget everything... and I mean everything... that mainstream medicine has told you about testosterone.

You see, losing your sex drive in your middle-age and senior years isn't all that unusual. Starting around age 30, your levels of testosterone — the key male sex hormone — start to take a nosedive.

And by the time you reach 60 or so, you may only be producing a fraction of the testosterone that you were making in your 20s.

So the solution is simple, right? Just replace the testosterone you're losing, and your sex drive will come roaring back to life.

But, unfortunately, many guys I treat are scared to start testosterone treatments because they've been told that testosterone could cause a heart attack.

You may have heard the same thing… maybe even from our own government. And I'll tell you what I tell my male patients.

Testosterone DOES NOT cause heart attacks… but some testosterone PRODUCTS may.

That's the truth, as straightforward as you'll ever hear anyone tell it.

You see, not too long ago the FDA required labels to be put on prescription testosterone products warning of an increased risk of heart attacks and strokes.

That scared the pants off a lot of guys — and I don't blame them. But it's only PART of the story as far as testosterone is concerned.

You see, the FDA based its move on a study of men over the age of 65 who were getting testosterone therapy. The guys getting testosterone were more likely to have heart attacks.

But here's where our government screwed up… BIG TIME!

The men in the study were taking a gel form of testosterone that you see advertised on TV — and they were taking HUGE doses of it.

Now, I could have told them before this study started how it was going to turn out. Because lots of experienced docs like me have learned to stay far away from these topical testosterone gels.

These gels are rubbed into your skin, and that's a problem. There's a significant amount of something called "aromatase enzyme" in your skin, and it causes testosterone to be converted into estrogen.

Yes, you read that right — estrogen. And high estrogen does increase the risk of heart attacks in men, along with increasing your chances of prostate enlargement and growing breasts.

In other words...

It's not the testosterone causing heart attacks... *it's the estrogen.*

And even if the testosterone makes it past your skin without being converted into estrogen, it can still run into problems in the hair follicles that cover your body.

There's an enzyme in the hair follicle called 5 alpha reductase which turns testosterone into DHT. The problem with too much DHT is that it causes prostate enlargement, hair loss where you don't want it (like your head) and hair gain where you might not want it (like your back).

It also can make your testicles shrink — and no guy wants that.

The only reason these testosterone gels are pushed on guys is that Big Pharma can charge up to $300 a month.

It's a scam... and one that's giving testosterone a bad name.

But doctors like me — ones who aren't in the drug companies' pockets — have been safely using testosterone injections and sublingually (under the tongue) for years. And the results I see time and time again include:

- Huge boosts in sex drive;
- Improvements in sexual performance (including reversing erectile dysfunction);
- Weight loss and muscle gain;
- A better mood and less irritability;

- Less brain fog and improved concentration; and
- Energy surges like you haven't felt in years.

And the science — when it doesn't involve massive doses of testosterone gels — proves that testosterone replacement therapy is safe and may even add quality years to your life.

Not too long ago, a study looked at testosterone replacement therapy in the VA hospital system.

Researchers followed 83,000 male veterans for 14 years. The guys who got testosterone replacement were 47 percent less likely to die, 18 percent less likely to have a heart attack, and had 30 percent fewer strokes.

Testosterone actually REDUCED your chances of heart attack or stroke!

A couple of other studies were reported as abstracts at an American Urological Association meeting.

One looked at men with type II diabetes and had 340 subjects that were given injected testosterone.

The results showed that glucose levels improved, hemoglobin A1C levels improved, triglycerides were reduced in the blood, blood pressure dropped, and erectile function improved.

So for diabetics, as we've always known, testosterone can be very good. This was a long study, too, with 87 months of treatment.

Another study of 262 patients using testosterone showed weight loss, a decrease in total cholesterol, an increase in HDL (good) cholesterol, improved glucose levels and prostate symptom scores improve significantly.

So what's the lesson here? Testosterone therapy, when it's done correctly, is extremely low risk and potentially life-changing for millions of guys.

But you need to find a doc who knows what he's doing. Remember, the mainstream docs who prescribe gels have basically been trained by the drug companies.

Some drug rep comes into the physician's office and tells him how to prescribe the gel and the doctor starts writing prescriptions. The doctors don't take the time to educate themselves or learn how to provide testosterone therapy safely and effectively.

Always look for a doctor who only does testosterone injections or sublingual administration and don't be afraid to ask him about his experience and the results he's seen.

Because, in the right hands, testosterone treatment can help eliminate the need for erectile drugs, diabetes medicines, high blood pressure pills, antidepressants and the plethora of other drugs the mainstream medicine tries to cram down our throats.

THE FEMALE SEX DRUG YOU SHOULD NEVER BUY

Let's face it — sexual dysfunction isn't just a problem guys face with age.

There are millions of older women out there who just aren't "in the mood" any more, and who don't get that urge for sex like they used to.

But be careful — because if you go to your typical mainstream doctor's office with this problem, you could be in for the disappointment of a lifetime.

Because there's a drug on the market now that promises to improve female libido, and it may be…

The greatest sexual health scam EVER perpetuated on women!

In 2015, the FDA voted to approve a new drug that's being called the "Viagra for women." It's called flibanserin, and it's sold under the brand name Addyi.

You see, flibanserin isn't some revolutionary, life-changing drug. It's the very definition of a dud, and I won't prescribe it to patients.

Flibanserin had been before FDA panels twice previously

— and both times it was voted down.

And that made sense, because this drug has numerous side effects that include increasing the risk of fainting and some potentially serious drug interactions.

Even worse? It doesn't work very well.

In the clinical trials, there was only around 10 percent efficacy. Or, in other words…

You'd have to treat 10 women for ONE to benefit!

That's outrageous! The other 9 would be completely out of luck, but they'd still be exposed to all the potential side effects.

And flibanserin is a drug you have to take every day… whether you want to have sex or not.

So it's perfect for the drug companies — and not so great for you.

And how did this drug ever see the light of day to begin with? Well, that's the most shameful part of the story.

Drug companies have been chomping at the bit ever since Pfizer did a study years ago that found that 63 percent of women suffer from sexual dysfunction. Now that's what I call a huge market!

Unfortunately, Pfizer's drug, Viagra, didn't work for women… so other companies started taking their turn. That's how flibanserin turned up.

There was even a simple, five-question screening tool developed to determine which women should get the drug.

See how easy it is to end up on a medication for the rest of your life? So in other words, drug companies invented the disease and told doctors how to make the diagnosis.

Worse still, Big Pharma worked with women's groups and got them all riled up, claiming there were 26 different approved drugs to treat men's sexual dysfunction and none for women.

They made this about equal rights… and not about

whether flibanserin works at all!

That's shameful! One congresswoman even wrote the FDA and demanded the agency approve the drug — efficacy be damned!

What we already know about flibanserin is bad, and I predict it's going to get a whole lot worse.

Flibanserin is actually a failed antidepressant that lowers serotonin and increases dopamine and norepinephrine. These are our neurotransmitters and they are very carefully balanced in our nervous systems.

Drug companies indiscriminately alter the neurotransmitter levels without having a clue about what they're doing. That's a recipe for disaster.

To me this shows that the FDA is spineless and has very little regard for people's health.

I'm not saying that female sexual dysfunction isn't a problem. But I believe a holistic approach, and not taking a mind altering drug for the rest your life, is a much better way to deal with it.

Keep reading for natural treatments — including a delicious tea — that can jumpstart your libido without exposing you to the risks of potentially dangerous drugs.

5 DRUGS THAT DESTROY YOUR SEX DRIVE

When you start losing your sex drive, it can be easy to chalk it up to getting older.

We're conditioned to think that it's just a normal part of aging, and lots of us stop looking for answers completely.

But what if I told you that rekindling your sexual urges at any age could be dead simple? The problem may start with that medicine cabinet of drugs you're taking every day.

Lots of us don't read the fine print about the side effects of the drugs we're taking. But the fact is, there are countless drugs that can absolutely devastate your sex drive.

And getting these drugs out of your life can be the first step to enjoying the type of sexual desire you haven't felt in years.

Here are 5 drugs you should talk to your doctor about if you feel like your libido is down in the dumps.

Sex Killer #1: Antidepressants

Mainstream medicine hands out selective serotonin reuptake inhibitors (SSRIs), like Paxil, Prozac, and Zoloft, like candy.

But the same neurotransmitters they affect also play a key role in sexual desire and performance. Anywhere from 30 percent to 80 percent of people on these drugs end up facing problems in the bedroom.

Sex Killer #2: Allergy meds

Antihistamine drugs like Benadryl have been linked to a loss of sex drive. The effect is supposed to be temporary, but it's not that simple.

If you suffer from bad allergies, you may be taking these drugs nearly daily for months at a time. You're talking about a major hit to your sex life, and you may never even realize that your medications are causing it.

Sex Killer #3: Beta blockers

Drugs for high blood pressure are notorious for killing your sex drive — and, in fact, beta blockers come with a laundry list of other side effects like dizziness, weakness, fatigue, and diarrhea (none of which are great for a healthy sex life).

Some of the more common beta blockers on the market include Acebutolol (Sectral), Atenolol (Tenormin), Bisoprolol (Zebeta), and Metoprolol (Lopressor, Toprol-XL).

Sex Killer #4: Opioid painkillers

This is another class of drugs that the mainstream is prescribing like crazy for every ache and pain. In fact, the over-prescription of opioids like Vicodin and Oxycontin has become a national epidemic.

But, in addition to making you feel like a zombie, opioids can lower your testosterone levels. And nothing kills sex drive faster than Low T.

Sex Killer #5: Benzos

Benzodiazepine drugs like Xanax and Valium are often given to help with anxiety. But, like opioids, they can leave you feeling like a zombie and can destroy your sex drive.

Plus, major medical groups have advised against prescribing benzos to most seniors, because their side effects and risks often outweigh their benefits.

If you're taking any of these drugs and are experiencing loss of sexual desire, make an appointment with your doctor right away. Talk about switching to meds with a lower risk profile — and see whether there are lifestyle changes or natural supplements that can get the same results.

You'll find many of them throughout this book.

THE SECRET "SEX TEA" HUSBANDS AND WIVES CAN SHARE

Earlier in this chapter I talked about the "female Viagra" drug — and how it's a dud that is absolutely useless for most women.

But let's be honest — you ladies really have been getting a raw deal for years.

There are millions of guys carrying around "little blue" erection pills in their wallets… and Big Pharma can't come up with a single good treatment for women.

But where the drug companies have failed, Mother Nature has answered the call.

Because growing in the high peaks of the Andes Mountains in Peru is a…

Powerful sexual BREAKTHROUGH that works for both men AND women!

I'm talking about the maca plant — and its root has been used in traditional folk medicine for hundreds of years.

Now we've learned that maca root is a powerful libido booster that can jumpstart your sex drive in just weeks!

And this natural remedy doesn't care about your gender.

According to Dr. Hyla Cass, "In my practice, I have seen maca restore hormonal imbalance and related sexual desire and fertility in both men and women."

Maca root is rich in fatty acids and amino acids, which are both critical to a healthy sex life. Plus, maca root seems to act as an adaptogen (like rhodiola and ashwagandha), which means it helps to calm stress and balance hormone levels.

And balancing your hormones is a critical first step in addressing sexual dysfunction.

In a massive analysis on previous studies of maca root, researchers found that both men and women reported major increases in their sexual desire. In fact...

They started seeing results in as little as 14 days!

Could you really be just two weeks from the best sex you've had in years?

In another 8-week study, men who took just 1,500 to 3,000 mg of maca root a day also experienced significant increases in sexual desire.

And clinical studies have found that it both improves sexual desire and decreases menopause symptoms in women... the types of symptoms that can kill your sex drive fast.

Even the University of Michigan admits that "Maca appears to be beneficial in treating menopausal symptoms."

If you haven't heard about the wonders of maca root before, believe me, it's not your fault. Big Pharma and the mainstream medical establishment have no interest in allowing a natural remedy to take a chunk out of the billion-dollar sexual dysfunction market.

But if you're interested in giving maca root a try, it couldn't be easier. You can pick up maca 1,600 mg capsules at **www.pipingrock.com**.

And here's an even better idea. You can actually pick

up maca root in powdered form, which can be added to a delicious tea or smoothie.

It's a romantic drink you can enjoy with your partner before a night of romance.

You can pick up maca powder from companies like Organika at **www.luckyvitamin.com.**

THIS ED REMEDY IS SO POWERFUL, BATTLES WERE FOUGHT OVER IT!

You won't read about it in most history books… but in 1685, a major skirmish broke out along the Chinese-Korean border.

Arrows were fired… men were killed and wounded.

And the Chinese emperor was so furious that he ordered all the Korean perpetrators (and even the local political officials) executed!

They weren't fighting over gold… or water… or farming land. This battle was over…

The most powerful, natural ED fighter on the planet!

I'm talking about Korean red ginseng (often called Panax ginseng). And if you suffer from erectile dysfunction, it could hold the secret to ending those embarrassing nights and performance problems forever.

In traditional Asian cultures, Korean red ginseng has been prized for its healing powers — and as a sexual stimulator — for centuries.

Now we know that this powerful plant, which grows all across Asia, can be a powerful weapon in the fight against ED.

In a study out of Korea, published in the prestigious *Journal of Urology*, men with ED took 900 mg of Korean red ginseng three times a day — or a placebo — for 8 weeks.

And the results were unbelievable!

Nearly two-thirds of men taking Korean red ginseng reported significant improvements in their ED symptoms. And these were differences the guys (and their partners) felt in the bedroom.

Men taking Korean red ginseng reported big improvements in their ability to maintain an erection and achieve penetration during sex.

Medical scans even PROVED that these men were achieving better, firmer erections than before.

So tell me — what would those kinds of results mean for you?

The secret to Korean red ginseng appears to be compounds called ginsenosides, which can relax the muscles of the penis and encourage blood flow.

And even the esteemed Mayo Clinic has testified to how remarkably safe Korean red ginseng is. It doesn't come with the kinds of side effects you see from prescription ED pills like Viagra or Cialis.

Plus, this wasn't the only study that proved Korean red ginseng could help you ditch your annoying ED issues for good.

A huge analysis of previous studies on Korean red ginseng, published in 2008, found that it produced a "significant effect" in relieving ED.

And because of Korean red ginseng's excellent reputation, getting your hands on it couldn't be easier.

You can pick up NOW Foods Panax Ginseng for about $10 a month at **www.puritan.com.**

CHAPTER SEVEN

HEAL YOUR HEART WITH THESE SIMPLE (AND SAFE) TRICKS

REVERSE YOUR HEART DISEASE IN 5 EASY STEPS

It was one of my father's favorite sayings — the definition of insanity is doing the same thing over and over again and expecting a different result.

And let me tell you something…

The way we're treating heart disease in this country is ABSOLUTELY INSANE.

Let me prove it to you…

HALF of the world's bypass and stent procedures are performed in Americans… and about 30 percent of adults over the age of 40 are taking a cholesterol-lowering statin.

And all these pills and surgeries haven't accomplished a darned thing.

We still have the highest rate of heart disease in the world, and **cardiovascular deaths are actually INCREASING again.**

That doesn't shock me. Research has shown that statins don't extend lives — and neither do angioplasties, stents, and coronary bypass surgeries.

But what does shock me is that the mainstream keeps recommending the same pills and procedures OVER. AND.

OVER. AGAIN.

Like I said… it's insane.

But today is the day we get you off this merry-go-round forever.

Because I'm going to introduce you to the 5-step heart health protocol I recommend to my own patients.

It can help stop blood clots, prevent heart attacks, and even reverse heart failure.

And the best part? You won't need ANY prescription drugs or surgeries.

Heart Healer #1: Get Plenty of Sunlight

There are few things in nature that get a bad rap more than the sun, yet this villainized energy source is a key player in your health — especially heart health.

In fact, if you don't get enough sun on your skin every day, you're missing out on the easiest — and by far, the cheapest — way to reduce your risk of cardiovascular disease.

A large study published last year in the *Journal of Internal Medicine* set out to determine if sun exposure had any impact on your risk of dying from cardiovascular disease.

Boy did it ever!

The researchers found that **women who got regular sun exposure lived an average of 1 to 2 years longer** than those who didn't. One key reason for this was because they had a significant decrease in cardiovascular disease events, such as heart attacks and stroke.

Light frequencies from the sun activate the production of sulfated cholesterol in the skin.

This compound plays an important role in preventing the type of blood clotting that can trigger a heart attack or stroke.

Sulfated cholesterol also…

- Keeps our red blood cell membranes intact so that they can squeeze through the tiny capillaries in our circulatory systems;
- Helps repair damage of the inner lining of our arteries; and
- Is water-soluble, which means it can easily travel to all tissues of the body.

Sulfated cholesterol also becomes sulfated vitamin D, which further reduces your risk of cardiovascular disease.

Heart Healer #2: Magnesium

It would be hard for me to overstate the importance of magnesium in heart health.

Magnesium is at the core of most of the enzymes that are involved in energy production. And energy production is critically important for tissues with a high-energy need, especially the heart muscle.

Magnesium has also been shown to inhibit blood clots, block calcium uptake, thin the blood, and relax the blood vessels — many of the very things prescription drugs are supposed to do!

Low magnesium is associated with elevated blood pressure, which is a risk factor for cardiovascular disease such as heart attacks and strokes.

At one point in time, we were able to get all the magnesium we needed in magnesium-rich foods like leafy vegetables, nuts, legumes, whole grains, fish, and fruits.

Unfortunately, the magnesium content of food has been declining in recent years — a problem that is only compounded by the fact that 80 to 95 percent of total magnesium is removed in the processing of grains.

As a result, most Americans don't get anywhere near the recommended daily allowance of 400 mg of magnesium.

This means that most of us would benefit from magnesium supplementation.

There are various forms of magnesium supplements, but you have to choose carefully because a lot of them aren't well-absorbed by the body. My favorite is magnesium threonate, which is a more recent formulation that has been shown to penetrate the mitochondrial membrane and the blood-brain barrier.

Heart Healer #3: Coenzyme Q10

No heart disease protocol would be complete without coenzyme Q10. Many studies show that CoQ10 supplementation can reduce the risk of cardiovascular disease, improve heart function, and can even prevent brain degeneration.

It's also been shown in studies to help reverse the symptoms of heart failure.

Like magnesium, CoQ10 plays a role in energy production, which is critical for heart health. It is involved in electron transfer to create energy in our "tiny energy factories" called the mitochondria.

As with many other nutrients, CoQ10 levels decline with aging, which makes supplementation even more important.

For those over 50, I recommend the ubiquinol form of CoQ10 (rather than ubiquinone). Ubiquinol is better absorbed through the gastrointestinal tract and acts more efficiently in the mitochondria to improve energy in our cells.

Heart Healer #4: DHA

Another critical component for reducing cardiovascular risk is the omega-3 fatty acid DHA, which is abundant in seafood, especially cold water fish.

DHA is a special molecule in nature that transmits

electric and light signals and is present in all high-energy tissues in animals.

Studies show that low levels of DHA greatly increase the risk of cardiovascular disease. And there's nothing that depletes our bodies of DHA more than eating processed food.

You can supplement with DHA, but I prefer getting my DHA from my diet. DHA is abundant in low-mercury fish like wild-caught salmon, sardines, trout, and cod. It's also present in shellfish, which has the added benefit of containing sulfur, which is needed for the sulfation of cholesterol and vitamin D.

Heart Healer #5: Vitamin K2

Getting enough vitamin K2 could be a matter of life and death when it comes to heart health.

The Rotterdam Heart Study of nearly 5,000 people showed that participants that ingested the greatest quantities of vitamin K2 in their diet *experienced a 57 percent reduction in death from heart disease compared to people who ingested the least.*

The reason why vitamin K2 is such a critical factor in heart health is because it helps keep calcium from building up in your arteries.

Calcium is beneficial for your bones, but deadly for your arteries because it contributes to the buildup of plaque, which restricts blood flow to the heart.

Vitamin K2 makes sure calcium goes where it's supposed to: in your bones, and out of your arteries.

That's why, whenever my patients have a coronary artery CT scan that indicates an increase in deposition of calcium in soft tissues, I always recommend supplementing with vitamin K2.

There are two types of vitamin K2: MK-4 and MK-7.

MK-4 is found in certain animal foods, like goose liver pate, egg yolks, the dark meat of chicken, and raw, grass-fed dairy. The problem with MK-4 is that it only stays in the body for a few hours.

MK-7, on the other hand, stays in your system for days. It is found in fermented foods like natto (a fermented soy product used in Japan), and in certain cheeses like Swiss Emmental, Dutch Edam, French Brie, and Jarlsberg from Norway.

I recommend taking a supplement that contains both MK-7 and MK-4, with the total dose of at least 100–200 µg per day of total vitamin K2.

THIS HEART DISEASE IS DEADLIER THAN CANCER! (HERE'S HOW TO BEAT IT)

Most people I know are scared to death of getting cancer — and rightfully so. They hear the word cancer and think "death sentence."

But there's something out there more fatal than cancer — and it's on the rise in the U.S.

I'm talking about heart failure.

According to a recent study published in the *European Journal of Heart Failure*, heart failure is more fatal than the most common types of cancer.

And by a huge measure.

Just 5 years after diagnosis, men with heart failure had a 64 percent greater risk of dying than men with prostate cancer. And women with heart failure had an 82 percent greater risk of dying than women with breast cancer.

This was no small study, either. It examined data from more than 56,000 people over an 11-year period.

Contrary to its name, heart failure does not mean your heart has failed altogether.

Heart failure occurs when the heart isn't pumping as

well as it should be. The most obvious signs are shortness of breath and fatigue.

The reason heart failure is so deadly is because it doesn't just impact your heart — it impacts your entire body. That's because it's your heart's job to deliver oxygen- and nutrient-rich blood to the body's cells.

Poor pumping means the body's cells aren't getting enough blood — and this includes the cells in all of your major organs. When they don't get enough oxygen and nutrients, they eventually break down.

One key underlying reason for heart failure is something your doctor has likely never even talked to you about: your mitochondria.

Mitochondria are our cells' powerhouses. They're responsible for converting the food you eat into usable energy that powers every single cell in your body.

The problem is that as we get older, mitochondria become damaged and don't function as well, and they also decrease in number.

This creates a critical energy deficiency that has been connected to virtually all degenerative diseases, including — you guessed it — heart failure.

The good news is that you can take proactive steps to improve both your mitochondria and your heart function.

Following my 5-step heart protocol (discussed earlier in this chapter) is great for shielding your heart against all sorts of diseases. But if you have (or are worried about) heart failure, a few more steps may be in order:

- First, eat foods that are rich in electrons, such as healthy fats and fish. Your body actually strips the electrons from this food and delivers them to your mitochondria.

- Take a daily probiotic. This maintains a diverse microflora in your gut, which helps with the energy transfer from your food to your mitochondria.
- Have your testosterone and DHEA levels checked. I always test these levels on my patients with heart failure. If they're low, bringing them up improves heart function.
- Last but not least, numerous supplements have been shown to help heart failure. Some of the most potent include CoQ10 (as discussed earlier), hawthorn berry, carnitine, D ribose, and the amino acid taurine.

[WARNING] THESE POPULAR ANTIBIOTICS DOUBLE YOUR RISK OF ANEURYSM

I don't care how many years you've been practicing medicine or how tough you think you are.

Having a patient die is still a painful and emotional experience.

And it's a lot worse when you know that patient's death could have been prevented.

One of my patients, Tom, came within moments of dying not too long ago — and his story could save your life or the life of someone you love.

You see, Tom had been admitted to a hospital with pneumonia, when another doctor gave him a prescription for Levaquin, a common antibiotic.

A few months later, he developed a dissection (a type of tearing) in the aorta, one of your body's main arteries. It took emergency surgery to barely save Tom's life. But, believe it or not, Tom isn't alone.

He was just the latest victim of a class of antibiotics called fluoroquinolones, which have left people broken, in pain, and fighting for their lives.

We've known about the incredible dangers of fluoroquinolones for years. But, believe it or not, your risk of ending up on one of these antibiotics is now greater than ever.

Getting "Floxxed"

The Food and Drug Administration doesn't have the backbone to pull fluoroquinolones off the market.

But the FDA has still sent a pretty strong message about these drugs — it doesn't want you or anyone you know taking them.

I'm dead serious. Let me explain.

The fluoroquinolones on the market today include:

- Avelox (moxifloxacin);
- Cipro (ciprofloxacin);
- Floxin (ofloxacin);
- Levaquin (levofloxacin);
- Noroxin (norfloxacin); and
- Tequin (gatifloxacin).

You'll notice that all of their generic names are pretty similar and include "flox." That's because these drugs are all basically knock-offs of each other.

And they harm so many people that there's become a term for it in the medical community: "Getting floxxed."

The problem got so bad with so many people "getting floxxed" that even the government had to step in and take action.

In 2008, the FDA slapped a black-box warning on fluoroquinolones, after a lawsuit by a citizen's group revealed that *they were causing tendons to rupture.*

But the problems didn't stop there… not by a longshot.

You see, fluoroquinolones damage tendons because they

attack the collagen. That means they can attack collagen anywhere in your body… including your arteries.

A recent study showed that you **DOUBLE your risk of an aortic aneurysm,** where a bubble can develop on the artery, if you've had a recent course of a fluoroquinolone antibiotic.

These aneurysms are usually a death sentence — and the problem can start in as little as 60 days after starting on fluoroquinolones.

There has been evidence of other possible effects of fluoroquinolone antibiotics, including:

- Cardiac dysrhythmias;
- Peripheral nerve damage;
- Myasthenia gravis (an autoimmune disorder that affects the muscles);
- Aortic rupture;
- Fibromyalgia;
- Vision and hearing loss;
- Anxiety;
- Hallucinations; and
- Chronic fatigue.

The fluoride in these drugs acts as a toxin, and damages our mitochondria — the energy centers for our cells. It also lowers the ability of the water inside our cells to transmit energy.

And when you start messing around with mitochondria and cellular function, you're inviting all kinds of degenerative diseases to take hold.

Unsafe at Any Dose

So many people have been harmed by fluoroquinolones… so many folks have gotten "floxxed"… that last year the

FDA did something you almost never see.

The agency released a SECOND black-box warning, and this one wasn't messing around.

It basically said… **Don't take fluoroquinolones under ANY CIRCUMSTANCES, unless there are no other alternatives.**

That's about as clear language as you're ever going to see. Even our government — which is deep in Big Pharma's pockets — does not want very many people taking these meds.

And, still, **33 MILLION prescriptions** for fluoroquinolones are being written every single year!

That's greater than the entire population of Texas!

How on Earth is this happening? Why are doctors putting so many people are risk?

Well, there are two things going on here… and neither one of them is good.

> **Problem #1:** Doctors are ignoring the warnings. It may sound hard to believe, but I've found that doctors routinely ignore FDA warnings. So they wouldn't think twice about prescribing fluoroquinolones.
>
> Making the problem worse, lots of times these drugs are prescribed for no good reason at all. They're handed out for illnesses they can't treat, like sinus infections, colds, or bronchitis. Studies have shown that 30 percent to 50 percent of antibiotic prescriptions may be unnecessary.
>
> So you're getting all of the risk, for absolutely no benefit.
>
> **Problem #2:** The bacteria in our bodies build up resistance to certain antibiotics, so doctors need to experiment with new ones (including

ones that may be riskier). This is a well-known consequence of the over-prescribing of antibiotics that's been going on for years.

If you're prescribed a fluoroquinolone antibiotic, odds are it's because of Problem #1 and not Problem #2. That's why you need to advocate for yourself.

Talk to your doctor about whether you really need the antibiotic in the first place. And, if you do, see if you can switch to something safer.

THE DEVILISH DUO THAT'S DAMAGING YOUR HEART

The numbers are enough to make your head spin.

There's a heart attack every 34 seconds in America... and a death related to heart disease every minute.

Heart disease is a full-blown epidemic. And what does the Centers for Disease Control and Prevention recommend?

The same stuff you've heard a million times... stay on your meds, cut the fat and cholesterol, eat lots of fruits and veggies, exercise, and don't smoke.

Really revolutionary, huh?

But, listen, these are the same recommendations they've been making for years, and they haven't put a dent in the problem.

The fact is, there are major contributors to heart disease that our government hasn't begun to understand.

I call them the "devilish duo" — artificial light and man-made electromagnetic fields. And if you can limit your exposure to both, you'll be well on your way to...

Stopping deadly heart disease before it EVER develops!

I have to warn you… this area of medicine is controversial.

There are powerful industries, including the utility companies and the telecommunications giants that have been trying to squash it for years. They want you to believe, for example, that it's safe to roll out an explosion of man-made, electromagnetic fields (EMFs) that are up to 1 million times greater than the native EMF around the planet Earth.

Of course, that's nonsense… and I've seen the proof with my own patients. Let me prove it to you.

First, let's start with artificial light (especially blue light).

In 1924, Paris was lit up with electric lights. We humans have progressively and continually lit up more of our environments.

Basically, we have switched from outdoor to indoor creatures. But, unfortunately, our biology hasn't changed.

Research in this area is clear. Artificial light, and particularly the blue spectrums of that light, immediately destroys melatonin.

Melatonin is a hormone produced in the pineal gland of the brain and is secreted starting as the sun goes down and increases for about three hours before we go to bed.

Melatonin makes us sleepy so that we can fall asleep when we go to bed. Without natural darkness, melatonin levels do not rise which can lead to insomnia or other sleep disorders.

But melatonin is responsible for more than a good night's sleep.

Melatonin is important for our immune system and is also a powerful antioxidant.

Many studies show that shift workers, that's people who work at night and are continually exposed to artificial blue light, have far greater incidence of diseases like heart disease and stroke.

Studies also show that a person that works at night **reduces their lifespan by about 6 years from this exposure.** Artificial light is also correlated to elevated cancer risk, diabetes, obesity, depression and sleep disorders.

So what can you do to reduce your risk of artificial light decreasing your melatonin levels, disrupting your circadian rhythm, and harming your health?

I recommend for my patients to get sun exposure in the morning between 6 AM and noon. Exposure at this time sets circadian timing in the suprachiasmatic nucleus of the brain better than any other method.

The suprachiasmatic nucleus is a collection of neurons located in the hypothalamus and is the master clock that controls circadian rhythm. The sun exposure should be done with adequate skin and eye exposure without sunscreen or sunglasses.

So how do you keep artificial light from wrecking your health?

I try to limit exposure to lights for approximately 3 hours before going to bed. This includes computer monitors, handheld devices, televisions and indoor lighting.

There are computer and cell phone applications that can reduce or remove the blue spectrum, as this has been shown to significantly reduce harmful effects on melatonin.

Blue-blocking glasses can also be worn at night and special blue–reduced lighting is also available. Candles, kerosene lamps, fires or the moon do not have significant blue light so are considered safe.

In my practice, for anyone with heart disease risk factors, sleep disorders, obesity, autoimmune diseases or diabetes, I always recommend reducing blue light exposure at night and setting circadian rhythm in the morning by getting a natural sunlight.

This is a relatively easy experiment that you can do on

yourself. Decrease the blue light exposure for a couple of months and see if your sleep improves. You can also check your laboratory values before and after reducing artificial light.

The two measures that I pay the most attention to when doing this are the CRP high sensitivity, which is a measure of inflammation, and sulfated DHEA which is a hormone marker of interleukin 6, an inflammatory cytokine.

Other good tests are salivary adrenal stress index and salivary melatonin, although they more difficult to get your doctor to order.

And here's how EMFs are harming your heart...

Electromagnetic fields (EMFs) are present in the technologies we use today, from power lines to the electricity running through our homes to everyday appliances (especially energy efficient), cell phones, cell towers, broadcast towers, power lines, wireless, cars, computers, smart meters, Wi-Fi, wireless routers, baby monitors and other electronic devices.

In other words, EMFs are everywhere, and they're bad for our health.

These devices emit electromagnetic radiation that can penetrate and affect us, seriously compromising our health and disturbing our environment.

The electromagnetic field of the earth is known as the Schuman's resonance and has a frequency of about 8 hertz.

Are all these man-made frequencies drowning out the Earth's natural field? You may have heard of the recent drastic decline in honey bees with colony collapse disorder. Scientists did an experiment where they placed a cordless phone in the bee hive.

The next day, none of the bees had returned to the hive. The EMFs from the cordless phone disrupted their navigation system, one of many biologic effects of EMFs.

As much as 3 percent of the population are sensitive to

EMFs and get acute symptoms when exposed.

These people are like the human canary in the coal mine!

There have been studies showing increased heart dysrhythmias with EMF exposure.

A cell phone in the pocket on a belt may harm sperm DNA, resulting in misshapen sperm and impaired fertility in men. Laptop computers with wireless Internet connections can also damage DNA and sperm.

There's a consistent pattern of increased risk for malignant brain tumors with the use of mobile and cordless phones according to Dr. Hardell at Orebro University in Sweden. The use of wireless devices such as phones and laptops by pregnant women may alter brain development of the fetus.

EMF exposure has been linked in both animal and human studies to hyperactivity, learning and behavior problems. Other health effects include effects on memory, learning, behavior, attention, sleep disruption, cancer and neurological diseases like Alzheimer's disease.

I suggest that most people have their homes and work environments tested, especially if there are any health or energy problems in the person. This can be done by hiring a specialist that can come to your home or workplace and do the appropriate testing. The other option is to purchase or rent EMF meters to test yourself.

One of the best places to start when trying to reducing EMF exposure in your own environment is to evaluate where you sleep.

There shouldn't be any electrical appliances in the bedroom and no cell phones. If you must have a cell phone on at night, it is best to place it across the room as far away from your body as possible. It is ideal to have the electricity shut off to the bedroom and this can be done by installing a special circuit breaker.

I turn Wi-Fi off at night completely (you can use a timer

switch, like you do for holiday lights).

I also recommend evaluating other areas where you spend time at home and at work. Your car can be another significant exposure. I test cars before I buy.

Tips for safer cell phone use:

Children should only use a cell phone in an urgent situation and should never hold the phone to their head.

All calls should be a short as possible and preferably using a speaker phone or an air tube conducting headset

It is safer to carry cell phones in a case or a purse and they should not be carried in a pocket or in any area next to the body. There is generally more radiation from a cell phone on the backside versus the front. The Pong cell phone case has been shown to reduce exposure to microwave radiation.

It is much safer to use a cell phone when you have optimal reception. With each signal bar short of full reception there is several hundred times more energy emitted from the cell phone.

When making a call, don't put the cell phone next your head until the other person has answered.There is more radiation emitted by the cell phone in the beginning of a call.

It is best not to talk on the cell phone inside a car — the signal bounces around the inside, causing increased exposure.

The cell phone also sends out a stronger signal when inside the car when moving to maintain contact with the cell tower, increasing your exposure to microwaves. I always put my phone on airplane mode when getting in the car.

If you must put a cell phone up to your head, I recommend that you frequently switch sides to let the one side of your head and brain recover.

THE STATINS WARNING EVERY SENIOR NEEDS TO HEAR

I've spent the past 20 years trying to warn everyone I meet about the dangers of cholesterol-lowering statins.

And I'll tell you… sometimes it feels like rolling a boulder uphill.

Doctors are still handing statins out like candy and putting millions of patients at risk. And lots of these folks are never told that…

Statins probably won't save your life — but they could end it.

I've seen firsthand in my practice just how worthless — and completely unnecessary — statins can be.

I can't tell you how many patients I've treated who had so-called "high cholesterol" but NEVER developed heart disease.

And I've also seen people with supposedly low cholesterol who died of heart attacks.

Even the federal government is starting to admit that its war on cholesterol and fat was misguided (and stupid). But that statins train just keeps rolling…

First, you need to understand that these drugs are basically metabolic poison. They decrease cell energy, which is why so many people experience fatigue and even pain when they take them.

Even researchers (the ones who haven't been paid off by the drug companies) are starting to come around on my way of thinking.

Listen to the title of an article published in March 2015 in *Expert Reviews in Clinical Pharmacology:* "How statistical deception created the appearance that statins were safe and effective in primary and secondary prevention of cardiovascular disease."

The authors' conclusions in this paper were that statins did decrease cholesterol but they failed to significantly improve heart disease outcomes.

In other words, you get all the risk… for very little (if any) benefit.

A second report in the same journal was titled "Statins stimulate atherosclerosis and heart failure: pharmacological mechanisms." And it's every bit as bad as it sounds…

This study reported that statins lower coenzyme Q10 and decrease cell energy production (bad news for your heart, which needs a lot of energy).

They also inhibit the synthesis of vitamin K2 which prevents calcification of arteries and other soft tissues.

Finally, researchers also reported that the statins inhibit the biosynthesis of selenium-containing proteins which is thought to be an underlying cause of the epidemic of heart failure in this country.

So, basically, **statins aren't saving your heart… but they may be damaging it permanently.**

Statins are a mass poisoning of millions of people, and Big Pharma keeps pushing to get more and more folks on these drugs.

And how are they getting away with it? Because they've conned so many people into believing the high cholesterol myth.

The drug companies and the medical system have everyone trained to think that any cholesterol over 200 is a disease that needs to be treated with a drug.

Of course this is dead wrong, and many physicians and patients are beginning to realize this.

A person can be perfectly healthy with a cholesterol over 200 and there's absolutely no intervention that they need.

Most of the randomized trials using statin drugs for primary prevention showed no improvement in life expectancy. In fact, they may even be shortening lives.

Duke University researchers were looking at terminally ill people that were on statin drugs.

They were thinking, "Why should I give a medicine to prevent heart attacks to someone that has only one year to live?" They were actually looking for ways to save money.

That's actually a good point, so they did a study of people that had less than one year to live and were on statin drugs for their cholesterol.

Half were taken off of the drug and the other half were left on the drug. The results of the study are eye-opening and they were presented at the Annual Meeting of the American Society of Clinical Oncology.

First off, the patients taken off of the statin drugs lived almost **40 *days* longer** than those remaining on the drugs. Those taken off statins were also found to have a better quality of life, especially psychological well-being.

Hmmmm. That seems to support my hypothesis that statins are poisonous and shorten your life. They sure were poisonous in this study.

If you have heart disease with plaque in your arteries, especially if you've had stents or bypass surgery, your doctors will demand that you be on statins. That is also usually true if you're diabetic.

Why not look at better ways to decrease inflammation and protect your heart, like turmeric or curcumin supplements?

Instead, we have at least 8 different statin drugs approved in the United States and, believe it or not, the drug companies are continuing to introduce new ones.

It's because statins have been a cash cow for the drug companies — that's the reason we have so many versions of the same bad drug.

Let's see… 8 versions of the same poison. When it comes to health, money rules. Together we can change that.

THE POWER MINERAL THAT YOUR HEART ABSOLUTELY CRAVES!

There is a mineral that is incredibly important for our heart and brain health... that we'd literally die without... and it continues to be in short supply in our modern, processed food diet.

And that's terrible news for our health.

This wonder mineral is potassium, and it is critical for our nerves and hearts, and for fluid and electrolyte balance.

If our potassium goes too low, we die — simple as that.

A study published in the *Journal the American Medical Association, Internal Medicine,* with data from the National Health and Nutrition Examination Survey, found that people in the upper-quartile range for potassium were less likely to die or suffer heart attacks or strokes.

So one might ask, "How much potassium are we talking about here?" In the NHANES study, the lowest quartile of potassium intake was about 1.8 g a day and in the highest quartile the intake was about 4 g per day.

Now the mortality benefits with higher intake are very significant, up to a third less. So it looks as though we definitely want to try to get our intake at least to that level.

How easy is it to get at least 4 g of potassium daily in the diet? Would it be better to resort to potassium supplements?

First off, taking potassium supplements is usually not a good option as supplements are only allowed to have 99 mg of potassium.

So even if you took 10 tablets, you wouldn't even get 1 g of potassium.

As the NHANES data tells us, it's easy to have a low potassium intake if we eat the standard American diet full of refined grains, sugars and refined vegetable oils as there is very little potassium in these foods.

Root vegetables like beets, carrots and rutabagas are a very good source, having about 1.4 g per pound.

Green, leafy vegetables sources include spinach and kale, which can have up to 2.5 g per pound.

Winter squash and sweet potatoes are other good sources having about 2 g per pound.

There is also a good amount of potassium in meat and dairy products. I have a health program that I put patients on where I recommend a diet that consists of eating a lot of these foods.

Now there are other foods that are a good source of potassium that I don't recommend on a general basis for people who have chronic health problems.

One is bananas and another is oranges.

Everyone knows bananas are a rich source of potassium. The problem with bananas is that through hybridization, the banana is becoming a rich source of sugar and particularly fructose, which most of us cannot handle well.

Other foods that are relatively high in potassium but, in my opinion, should be limited in consumption in people with degenerative diseases are potatoes and tomatoes.

The bottom line — eating a natural foods diet with lots

of cooked vegetables, especially the root vegetables, will give you plenty of potassium.

A shot of organic carrot juice every day will pile on more potassium. Adding organic animal products such as meat and dairy round out a diet that will place you in the low-risk category as far as potassium intake is concerned.

$300 FOR FISH OIL?
THEY MUST BE CRAZY!

It's one of the dirtiest tricks in Big Pharma's arsenal.

And now they're targeting one of the safest and healthiest supplements around — fish oil.

The drug companies have been pushing for years to require any supplement that makes a health claim to do clinical trials.

Then the FDA comes in, bans all competing natural products that haven't done trials, and only allows the "tested" supplement made by the drug company to be sold. This system has already taken hold in Europe.

I could envision this happening with a drug like Lovaza, which is just a patented version of fish oil.

Fish oil has been shown to improve heart health. So a drug company took fish oil, did clinical trials, and made it into Lovaza.

I had a patient come up to me and say, "Hey Doc, I don't want to pay $20 a month for fish oil, can you write me script for Lovaza because my co-pay is $10."

So this guy is thinking, "I'll save $10 a month by getting

the prescription fish oil."

Pretty smart, actually, as this would add up to over $100 a year in savings for the patient.

But guess what? Lovaza costs $300 to $900 a month, a difference to regular fish oil only in price, not efficacy. I mean it's still just fish oil.

We all ultimately pay for this in the form of higher health insurance premiums. It really harms everyone except the pharmaceutical companies and their shareholders; oh yeah, and my patient who's saving $10 a month.

The next step in this devious plan will be for the FDA to ban all fish oil supplements that have not had clinical trials.

You see, the pharmaceutical companies pay the FDA to monitor their clinical trials. And then, they get rewarded for that payment by having their competitors banned from selling the product.

When you have a monopoly, you can charge whatever you want. Then your only alternative would be to squeeze your own fish; or shell out the ridiculously inflated price for the drug.

This is a situation I continue to monitor closely. They haven't banned fish oil yet, but trust me — it has a target on its back.

In the meantime, continue to stock up on quality fish oil from your local supplement shop or online. Buying Lovaza may make Big Pharma rich… but it won't do anything extra to protect your heart.

CHAPTER EIGHT

HOW TO BEAT DIABETES WITHOUT A PRESCRIPTION

REMARKABLE "QUEEN'S FLOWER" REVERSES DIABETES

When you learned that you had diabetes, you weren't just handed a diagnosis… you were handed a life sentence.

In fact, your doctor probably told you — in so many words — that life as you had known it was over.

Most diabetics are basically told the same three things by mainstream medicine:

#1: You have to swear off your favorite foods… including those delicious desserts… forever.

#2: You're going to have to take prescription medications (and sometimes several of them) for the rest of your life.

#3: Diabetes can't be cured — only managed.

But what if everything we've been told about diabetes is a bald-faced lie?

I'll tell you exactly what I've told countless diabetic patients who have come to see me over the years. Diabetes DOES NOT have to be a life sentence — or a death sentence.

You can get off of your meds, reverse your disease, and start living the healthy, diabetes-free life you deserve.

The secret is to stop treating your diabetes and start curing it.

You see, the mainstream treatments on the market today are just designed to treat your symptoms, and nothing more. They give you an insulin boost or help pull blood sugar out of your bloodstream.

But they don't do anything to treat the underlying cause of your diabetes in the first place — and that's why they can't cure it.

Alternative doctors have been a bit better, offering natural treatments like berberine and chromium. And I use both regularly in my practice.

But years ago, I discovered an amazing diabetes break-through from Asia — one that I've used to help reverse cases of diabetes that other doctors would have called hopeless. I'm talking about...

A powerful, natural diabetes fighter that even most alternative doctors don't know about!

It's called banaba leaf (sometimes known as "Queen's flower"), and it comes from one of the holiest and most legendary trees found in Southeast Asia.

The banaba tree produces beautiful leaves and flowers, and it thrives in Southeast Asia, India, and the Philippines. The people of Asia have been using banaba leaf in tea and to treat a variety of health conditions for ages.

Banaba is a remarkably revered tree in Buddhist culture. In one sect of Buddhism, it's considered to have played a key role in helping religious leaders attain enlightenment.

And banaba is an absolute breakthrough for the millions of people suffering from diabetes right now.

In fact...

This miracle plant attacks diabetes at the source, so you can REVERSE your disease!

Banaba isn't just some folk remedy without much science behind it. In fact, it's been the subject of dozens of studies from all around the world, going all the way back to 1940.

And its ability to improve even the worst symptoms of diabetes is remarkable. I've seen these results myself, time and time again.

Banaba extract contains a powerful compound called corosolic acid that works as an antioxidant and can lower blood sugar. In fact studies on corosolic acid from banaba have found that it **begins reducing blood sugar in as little as one hour!**

Corosolic acid activates proteins in your body that are responsible for transporting glucose from your bloodstream to your cells, where it belongs (this is how it lowers blood sugar).

Within **just two hours** of taking banaba extract with corosolic acid, people typically see a *10–15 percent reduction in their blood sugar levels.*

That can be enough to bring you into the normal range!

And banaba also works great for the long-term management of diabetes.

In one study on people with high blood sugar, patients reported a reduction of fasting glucose of nearly 17 percent — and their numbers were still down a year later!

And here's the best part...

There were absolutely NO side effects reported!

Imagine that — better blood sugar control without ANY of the side effects or risks that come with prescription diabetes meds. This is exactly why I've been recommending banaba to my own patients for years.

And in another, smaller study, patients were given either

32 mg or 48 mg a day of banaba extract, and after just two weeks they saw an average decrease of 30 percent in their blood glucose levels.

What's truly amazing about banaba is that it attacks your diabetes at the source, helping to improve many of the main health conditions that are contributing to the disease.

In fact, human and animal studies have shown that banaba works to reverse diabetes in at least 5 different ways…

> **Diabetes-Fighting Mechanism #1:** Banaba improves insulin sensitivity. In other words, it makes your cells less resistant to insulin, which is a major problem for diabetics. When insulin can do its job, you have less sugar in your bloodstream, where it can do damage.

> **Diabetes-Fighting Mechanism #2:** This powerful natural remedy increases your cells' ability to accept glucose, which is known as "cellular uptake." Your cells need glucose to operate correctly. And poor cellular uptake of glucose isn't just linked to diabetes — it can be a major risk factor for other degenerative diseases, like Alzheimer's.

> **Diabetes-Fighting Mechanism #3:** Banaba has been shown to lower cholesterol and triglyceride levels, which are main contributors to the heart disease that often accompanies diabetes. High cholesterol and triglycerides are extremely common among diabetics.

> **Diabetes-Fighting Mechanism #4:** Taking banaba extract can help you lose weight. Obesity is a major problem among diabetics, and is a main risk factor for the disease. If sugar isn't delivered to your cells,

it's going to be stored as fat. Fortunately, by helping your cells accept more glucose, banaba may help keep your weight in check. People have traditionally used banaba as a weight-loss aid, and animal studies have shown that taking banaba leads to less weight gain.

Diabetes-Fighting Mechanism #5: Banaba helps reduce oxidative stress and damage. Oxidative stress is a significant problem with diabetes, and leads to other health complications like heart disease and nerve damage. But banaba is a powerful antioxidant that has been shown to limit this type of damage.

So what kinds of results can banaba produce for folks like you? Just ask Rick, who had this to say in an online review.

"My blood sugar has consistently come down with continued use and has gone from a fasting 129 to a fasting 94 over the past year!"

Or how about Mary, who claims she lost 30 pounds in 3 months on banaba.

"I literally watched the pounds fall off," she wrote.

Banaba is a certified health miracle — one that attacks the root causes of your diabetes so you can enjoy your best blood sugar control in years.

And while many doctors still don't know about it, there are quality banaba supplements on the market that you can start taking right away.

You can buy Paradise Herbs Banaba Leaf for less than $20 a month at **www.iherb.com.**

THE GERMAN SECRET TO BEATING DIABETIC NERVE PAIN

If you suffer from type 2 diabetes, you know there's a lot more involved than just finger pricks, pills, and insulin shots.

The most frightening aspect of diabetes is all the health complications that come with it… things like heart disease, vision loss, poor circulation, and even memory problems.

And one of the most agonizing conditions that often accompanies diabetes is nerve pain… or what we doctors call peripheral neuropathy.

The nerve damage — which usually starts in your hands and feet — **can be absolutely excruciating.**

It can start with just a numbness, tingling, or a "pins and needles" feeling. But it can quickly lead to constant, round-the-clock pain that can make simple things like walking or sleeping nearly impossible.

Even the simple weight of a bed sheet or blanket can be incredibly painful if you're suffering from diabetic neuropathy.

And, if you're like a lot of diabetics, you've learned the hard way that even the most powerful prescription painkillers don't do a thing to ease this agony.

But the good news is that help is on the way. In fact…

Germany has had the answer for peripheral neuropathy for YEARS!

It's a natural compound called alpha lipoic acid, or ALA. ALA is a powerful antioxidant that I use in my own practice — and I've seen it work wonders on nerve pain and other symptoms of diabetes. And ALA has been an approved treatment for diabetic nerve pain in Germany for ages.

But with their obsession with handing our pricey prescription drugs, most American doctors have never tried it.

Much of the research on using ALA to treat peripheral neuropathy has focused on administering it intravenously — and that's an excellent way to quickly build up your body's levels.

A major study out of Germany looked at nearly 1,300 people with diabetic nerve pain, and the results were incredible.

After getting infusions of 600 mg a day for three weeks, patients saw major relief from their neuropathy. For example, they experienced:

- Less pain
- Decreases in prickling or burning sensations
- Improved sensation to stimuli, such as pinpricks and touch
- Better reflexes

That's right — **they began to reverse their diabetic nerve pain in just three weeks flat!**

Just consider how long you or someone you love has been suffering with the misery of diabetic neuropathy. What could these kinds of improvements — in just three weeks — mean for you and your quality of life?

And while, as I said, a great deal of the research on ALA

has focused on intravenous delivery, taking oral supplements can deliver results, too.

In one study published in 2006 in *Diabetes Care*, 181 patients with diabetic neuropathy took either oral ALA or a placebo for five weeks. And the folks on ALA experienced...

A whopping *50 percent more pain relief* than those taking placebo!

The patients saw the best results on about 600 mg of ALA a day.

So why is ALA so effective at reducing diabetic nerve pain? Well, as a powerful antioxidant, it hunts down and neutralizes dangerous free radicals throughout your body.

And these free radicals are a major culprit behind nerve damage and other complications that go hand-in-hand with diabetes.

Of course, the wonders of ALA don't end there. It's been proven in study after study to help your body use glucose more effectively and to improve insulin sensitivity.

That means **it fights your nerve pain and diabetes at the same time!**

An eight-week study out of Iran, published in 2011, found that patients who took ALA saw major improvements in insulin resistance and fasting blood glucose. They were literally reversing their diabetes!

I've seen ALA work absolute wonders for my diabetic patients, and I prescribe it regularly.

If you're interested in giving ALA a try, talk to your doctor about intravenous treatments. If he's unwilling to give them, find a doctor who will — the physician finder at the American College For Advancement in Medicine website (www.acam.org) is a great place to start.

You can also take supplements orally. Doctor's Best offers 600 mg Alpha Lipoic Acid supplements (the same dose used in research) that you can buy at **www.iherb.com.**

Remember, ALA is a natural antioxidant that you can find in fruits, vegetables, and even in our own bodies. But to get the kind of results you're looking for, you will need to supplement either intravenously or orally.

THIS HOUSEHOLD TIP COULD KEEP YOU DIABETES-FREE

It happens like clockwork every spring.

The local Orkin man… or some other pest-control company… starts coming around the neighborhood, promising to spray for bugs and make your home "critter-free."

And millions of us go for it, too.

Because, let's face it — nobody wants to see a line of ants on the kitchen counter or a silverfish scurrying across the basement floor.

But I'll tell you something… those professional bug zappers don't come around my house any more.

Because I operate by a pretty simple rule — and I hope you'll follow it, too.

I don't allow pesticides sprayed in my yard… in my home… or at my office.

Because the pesticides that are on the market today — even the pesticides that our government calls "safe" — are some of the most toxic chemicals on the planet. In fact…

Pesticide exposure can put you on the fast track to diabetes!

It's amazing that our government expects us to believe that the same chemicals that can kill ants, stinkbugs and cockroaches by the millions are perfectly healthy for us.

Of course, that's all a lie — and the research proves it.

There have been several studies over the years linking pesticide exposure to hormonal changes and chronic diseases, including diabetes.

In 2016, an international research team from England, Spain, and Greece attempted to pour through years of studies and data on pesticide exposure and diabetes, to see what it all said.

And what they found was truly frightening. They discovered rock-solid evidence that the following pesticides send your risk for developing diabetes through the roof:

- DDE (short for dichlorodiphenyldichloroeth-
  ylene — you'd better hope you never get that
  in a spelling bee);
- Heptachlor;
- Hexachlorobenzene (HCB);
- DDT (or dichlorodiphenyltrichloroethane); and
- Chlordane.

Now, when it comes to these pesticides (which belong to a family called organocholorines), there's some good news and bad news.

The good news is that most of them are already banned or restricted lots of places around the world, including in the U.S. But, like I said, there's bad news, too.

Bad News #1: If you were exposed to these pesticides before they were banned, there's a good chance they're still in your system. Plus, they're still in our soil and groundwater. They "bioaccumulate," which is a fancy way for saying they build up in our bodies over time. Studies done years after these pesticides were banned found that they were still present in Americans' bloodstreams. And they've been linked to diseases other than diabetes, including cancer and cognitive decline.

Bad News #2: These pesticides are likely just the tip of the iceberg. I'm not terribly convinced that the pesticides being used today are that much safer. At a minimum, they are toxins that produce systemic inflammation and hormonal changes, which are both contributors to degenerative conditions like type 2 diabetes.

So how can you protect your home — and your health?

First, follow my lead and don't use (or allow anyone else to use) commercial pesticides inside or outside your home.

There are actually perfectly safe and natural ways to keep bugs and other critters out of your home.

Keep in mind that for thousands of years, farmers didn't have access to these pesticide sprays. But they still had to keep insects and other nuisances from ruining their crops — or the farmers and their families would starve.

So you can go safe and low-tech like they did, to keep bugs away. Here's a recipe for an all-natural (and safe) pesticide.

Step #1: Mix three tablespoons of castile soap with one ounce of orange oil and one gallon of water.

Step #2: Shake the ingredients together vigorously.

Step #3: Pour the mixture into a spray bottle. This solution works especially well for slugs, ants and roaches.

The second thing I recommend is naturally detoxing to get these pesticides — and other unwanted toxins — out of your body.

Remember, as I said, pesticides "bioaccumulate" in your body and stay there. In fact, you'd be amazed how many toxins have built up in your system over the years, and may be contributing to your health problems.

The best way to help your body detox is by supporting your liver, which basically helps remove contaminants from your system.

Two truly effective liver supports are milk thistle and glutathione, which is a powerful antioxidant. You can buy 1,000 mg milk thistle capsules from Vitamin World at **www.vitaminworld.com.**

You can buy Jarrow Formulas glutathione in 500 mg doses at **www.puritan.com.**

A couple final tips — exercising and sauna treatments are both excellent ways to sweat toxins out of your body. And sweating is one of the best natural detox methods that we have.

And, finally, make the switch to organic produce whenever you can. And if you're not eating organic, make sure you wash your fruits and veggies thoroughly.

Remember that just because you cut out pesticides doesn't mean everyone else has. Pesticides are still found on much of the food we eat, and you want to keep as much of this poison as possible out of your body.

THE TERRIBLE ADVICE THAT'S MAKING YOUR DIABETES WORSE

If you're diabetic, you know it can wreak absolute havoc on your skin.

From dry, itchy patches to infections, you always seem to be dealing with one skin problem or another.

And once these issues start flaring up, mainstream doctors start handing out what I call...

The worst piece of advice ANY diabetic could get!

You may have gotten it yourself. At some point, a doctor may have advised you to limit your sun exposure or slather yourself with sunscreen any time you're outside.

That's not just terrible advice... it could actually be making your diabetes worse!

I'll tell you what I tell all of my patients — the sun is NOT our enemy. This is a crazy idea cooked up by a bunch of executives looking to sell billions worth of sunscreen.

And, unfortunately, the mainstream medical establishment bought it hook, line, and sinker.

I'm sure you've heard how important the sun is to helping your body make vitamin D — and vitamin D alone is protective against diabetes.

But, really, the benefits of the sun go much farther than that.

As I've explained throughout this book, sun exposure plays a critical role in stabilizing and optimizing your levels of key hormones, like melatonin.

And hormone balances can actually lead to the development or diabetes, or make existing diabetes worse.

In fact, researchers from Brigham and Women's Hospital in Boston have found that low melatonin levels are a major risk factor for diabetes.

And people with metabolic syndrome, a key precursor to diabetes, have consistently been found to have low melatonin levels.

The fact is, if you're diabetic — or looking to avoid diabetes...

Natural sun exposure is the best diabetes-fighting weapon you have!

Let me prove it to you.

In 2014, a research team from the University of Edinburgh in Scotland conducted an animal study that looked at key diabetes markers.

Mice that were regularly exposed to the kind of UV light you get from the sun:

- Were less likely to overeat
- Showed fewer signs of insulin resistance
- Had lower glucose readings

The scientists believe these benefits come from the nitric oxide that our skin produces when exposed to the sun. This nitric oxide has positive effects on our hormone levels, our metabolism, and our ability to manage our weight.

"We know sun-seekers live longer than those who spend

their lives in the shade," said Dr. Richard Weller, senior lecturer in dermatology at the University of Edinburgh. "Studies such as this are helping us to understand how the sun can be good for us."

Well, amen to that. I recommend more sun exposure to all... and I mean all... of my patients, and I can't tell you how quickly it begins to revitalize their health.

Here's my challenge for you.

I want you to focus on getting quality sun exposure each day — preferably starting in the morning — from now until your next doctor's appointment.

You're going to be shocked when you see things like your blood pressure and blood sugar start to decrease.

But I've seen it happen with countless patients. And I know it will happen for you, too.

IS BIG PHARMA GIVING YOU DIABETES IN A PILL?!?

When it comes to cholesterol-lowering statins, I feel like I've been living a bad dream for the past 30 years.

Big Pharma has sold a TRILLION dollars' worth of these poison pills — even though they come with life-wrecking side effects like:

- muscle pain;
- neuropathy;
- liver damage; and
- memory loss.

Just when you think the news on these drugs couldn't get any worse, it somehow does.

And if you're a woman serious about avoiding diabetes, you need to...

Read this before you swallow another statin pill!

A recent study showed that statins increase the risk of diabetes by *more than 50 percent* in older women.

After studying over 8,000 women aged 76–82 for 10 years, researchers found that the risk of new-onset diabetes increased by up to 51 percent in women taking statins.

That's right — new-onset diabetes.

That means these women weren't diabetic when they started taking statins — but they sure didn't stay that way.

In fact, the connection was so strong that the researchers conducting the study suggested that **older women avoid using higher doses of statins.**

I have a better idea: they should just avoid using statins altogether.

This isn't the first time statin use has been shown to increase the risk of diabetes.

A study published a few years back showed that women who used statins had a 71 percent elevated risk for diabetes compared to those not using statins.

Diabetes is nothing to mess around with. It is the leading cause of blindness, amputations, neuropathy, and kidney failure.

It also contributes to stroke and heart attack risk — an ironic twist, since statins are supposed to be protecting your heart.

By now, nobody should be surprised that statins are so harmful. After all, they "work" by lowering cholesterol — and cholesterol is absolutely essential for life!

You see, these meds were first developed for certain high-risk people, like those with genetic disorders that send their cholesterol numbers off the charts.

But in an effort to sell more pills, the drug companies have worked tirelessly to expand statins for prevention.

Don't fall for it.

Studies show that they don't save lives, which means that the risk simply outweighs the benefit.

The real answer for lowering heart risk and improving mortality is to get off processed foods, especially refined starches and vegetable oils.

It's not easy — especially at first — but it's effective. And in addition to lowering your risk of heart disease, you'll be lowering your risk of diabetes — and a host of other diseases — too.

CHAPTER NINE

ALL-NATURAL SOLUTIONS FOR PERFECT SLEEP

THE $10 SLEEP FIX THAT WORKS THE FIRST NIGHT (AND EVERY NIGHT AFTER)

If you suffer from trouble sleeping, you know it can wreak havoc on your health — and your quality of life.

How many night have you spent tossing, turning, staring at the ceiling, and just praying for a few hours of uninterrupted shut-eye?

And how many times have you had to suffer through a day groggy and unfocused, after a bad night's sleep?

Of course, turning to the mainstream medical establishment for help is practically useless. All they have to offer is sledgehammer sleeping pills that can leave you in a fog the whole next day — and that come with a list of side effects longer than your arm.

Well, your sleep troubles officially end today. Because I'm going to introduce you to…

A $10 sleep solution you'll feel working in MINUTES — and that you can rely on night after night.

This sleep fix is so effective that I use it myself — and so do my wife and children.

I can't wait to tell you all about it (it's going to seem a little strange). But before I do, let me give you the REAL reason you're having trouble drifting off to la-la land at night.

If you've researched sleep problems a bit, you may already be familiar with something called your circadian rhythm. It's like your body's internal clock, which tells you when you should be asleep and when you should be awake.

But what you may not know is that one of the ways we can seriously impair our health (and our sleep) is by upsetting our circadian rhythms.

And, unfortunately, that's become incredibly easy to do.

Our circadian rhythm affects our sleep/wake cycle, body temperature, blood pressure and the release of hormones.

Have you ever crossed multiple times zones and experienced jet lag? That's an example of your circadian rhythm being out of sync with where you are located on the planet.

And having a circadian rhythm that's out of sync can make you a sitting duck for sleep troubles and other serious, chronic diseases.

In fact, studies show that the night shift workers have increased rates of insomnia, cancer, cardiovascular diseases, metabolic syndrome, type 2 diabetes, obesity, low thyroid, and even fertility problems.

That's the bad news. The good news is that...

If you fix your circadian rhythm, you can fix your sleep problems and health — almost instantly.

Keeping your circadian rhythm healthy is all about light exposure, and getting on schedule with the Earth's 24-hour cycle.

First, you need to expose yourself to bright light on a daily basis.

Getting out in the morning sunshine has the most powerful effect on setting the optimal circadian rhythm for us. For example, going on a 20 minute walk in the morning, without sunglasses, is one of the best ways to keep your body and brain on the right schedule.

It's best to go outdoors several times a day, including in the late afternoon.

Another way to preserve optimal circadian rhythm is to avoid bright light at night and especially blue and white light (like the kind we get from computer and smartphone screens, and modern light bulbs).

Exposure to this kind of light at night basically tricks your body into thinking it's daytime.

And that's a big problem, because it leads to decreases in melatonin — a critical hormone that helps us stay asleep and keeps our immune systems working optimally.

Melatonin has powerful immune system benefits for both fighting infectious diseases and preventing cancer. Higher melatonin levels have been shown to help other health conditions too, like diabetes, glaucoma, hypertension, IBS and others.

Of course, you can take melatonin supplements, and sometimes I recommend them for patients. But it's far better to help your body make and keep melatonin naturally.

And to do that, you can try my…

$10 solution for PERFECT sleep — every night.

You want to limit your exposure to artificial light — such as blue light — at night. An easy way to do that is to shut off the TV, laptop, and phone, or to buy dimming programs like the f.lux software (which I use for my computer).

But a surefire way to stop artificial light exposure at night is with a simple pair of blue-light blocking glasses.

I've been using them for years, and have convinced my entire family to do the same. Even my college-aged son wears his blue-light blocking glasses at night to get great sleep.

These glasses shield you from artificial light, and help keep your circadian rhythm working properly. Even better, they stimulate the production of melatonin and keep your levels from falling off.

Start wearing them around 8 p.m. each night, and you'll notice something AMAZING happen (usually the first night). Within minutes, you'll start to feel more relaxed and sleepy — that's the melatonin kicking in.

And when you're ready for bed, your body will be prepared to give you the best night's sleep you've had in ages — absolutely no pills required.

This is a solution that works for people of any age. And blue-light blocking glasses are available everywhere online and are incredibly affordable.

I use Uvex glasses, which come in a range of styles and prices. I see Uvex Skyper glasses all the time on websites like eBay for around $10.

Just Google "blue light blocking glasses" and you'll have more choices than you can shake a stick at.

And remember — don't forget the kids and grandkids

Blocking blue light is just as important for the youngsters in our lives.

A study in *Pediatrics* evaluated 2,048 4th and 7th grade students in Massachusetts with the mean age of about 10 years.

The study showed that the children who had screened, electronic devices in their rooms had fewer minutes of sleep and later bedtimes. The kids with the devices had a full 20 minutes of less sleep on the weekdays than those that didn't.

Will 20 minutes of less sleep affect a kid? I think so.

There are some other simple things you can do to improve your quality of sleep, no matter your age, such as...

1. Having a steady, predictable bedtime;
2. Avoiding stimulating activities or substances in the evening;

3. Having a dark room with no night light or clock light because even a small amount of light can reduce melatonin production;

4. Utilizing some form of meditation or relaxation techniques; and

5. Avoiding eating heavy meals late in the evening.

COULD THAT SLEEPING PILL TURN INTO A NIGHTMARE?!?

You can't turn on the TV these days without seeing a commercial for some magic pill promising you the best sleep of your life.

And if you suffer from even occasional insomnia, asking your doctor for a prescription — or grabbing an over-the-counter sleeping drug — can seem like the answer to your prayers.

But this is where you need to be careful. Because as far as sleeping pills are concerned, many folks have found themselves in the middle of a real nightmare very quickly.

I'll explain more in a moment… but, first, it's important to understand a serious problem with how our government, through the Food and Drug Administration, approves these drugs.

In most cases, drugs are approved before the government and the manufacturer truly understand all the risks.

That's right…

Millions of Americans are guinea pigs… and they NEVER know it!

We might not know about serious reactions to a drug until a physician notices something unusual and publishes something known as a "case report."

I discovered an extremely alarming case report, published in the *Primary Care Companion for CNS Disorders* in August 2012 about two violent acts that were committed when a man and a woman were taking Ambien (the generic name of the drug is zolpidem) in combination with an SSRI antidepressant drug.

These were cases of violent murder that occurred in people without any previous violent history and they both claimed amnesia for the event.

One case was a 45-year-old man that stabbed his wife over 20 times in the middle of the night. The other was a 64-year-old woman that killed her husband with a crowbar while he was in bed.

In both of these cases, they had been taking zolpidem along with an SSRI antidepressant. Back in 2009 there was a case where a young man killed his girlfriend with a hammer striking her 40 times and his lawyers tried to blame the murder on the drug, the so-called Ambien defense.

My suspicion is that SSRIs can lead to violence on their own, but it might even be worse when taken along with zolpidem.

I know this sounds strange — but based on my experience with Ambien patients, I'm not terribly surprised.

I have seen many cases of patients who'd taken Ambien and reported weird dreams, sleepwalking, and eating at night, often with no recollection for it the next day.

They couldn't get off the stuff fast enough!

Then there was a patient I'll never forget, named Ted.

He got on Ambien after seeing a commercial that convinced him he should try it.

Within three days of taking Ambien, he went into a coma.

Three weeks later, and after a hospital bill of over $200,000 that included every scan and test known to man, the hospital doctors found nothing medically wrong with him.

They called it a reaction to Ambien, and the hospital physicians didn't report the event to the FDA. The FDA admits that less than 1 percent of all drug adverse reactions are actually reported.

Because of these risks, I prefer more natural sleep remedies.

You see, insomnia is a symptom of being out of balance, either emotionally or biochemically. Mainstream medicine's approach of trying to poison your way to health with drugs often ends in more problems, and sometimes with tragic results.

If you're taking a prescription or over-the-counter sleep-aid, talk to your doctor about getting off it as soon as possible. And keep reading this chapter for more ways to enjoy better sleep without resorting to potentially dangerous drugs.

4 STEPS FOR ERASING NIGHTTIME ANXIETY

We've all been there before.

It's late at night and you're tucked away in your bed. You're absolutely exhausted — but you just can't shut your brain off.

Your mind is racing with all the stresses and cares of the day. You keep replaying every anxious thought and worry, like a record player with the needle skipping.

Countless people suffer from nighttime anxiety, and it can make sleep nearly impossible.

Who can think about catching 40 winks when your heart is racing, you're short of breath, and your mind is on overdrive?

Whether you have a full-blown anxiety disorder — or just experience occasional anxiety attacks — there are plenty of things you can do to feel better (and get the good sleep you deserve).

Here are 4 natural (and drug-free) solutions for finally taming that evening anxiety for good.

1. Chamomile tea: The active ingredient in chamomile, apigenin, is known to bind to the same brain receptors as the active compounds found in drugs like Valium.

Chamomile is typically enjoyed as a tea, and studies have shown that long-term use can alleviate the symptoms associated with anxiety and other associated anxiety disorders. You can pick up chamomile tea at just about any supermarket. Brew a cup an hour or two before bedtime.

2. L-theanine is an amino acid found in green tea, and it may be the most relaxing natural substance around. You'll typically feel it working in just minutes.

L-theanine has been proven in clinical trials to relieve anxiety and the symptoms that are often associated with it. It can even help reduce blood pressure and a rising heart rate.

Because it's become a very popular supplement, L-theanine is very easy to get your hands on. You can pick up 200 mg bottles from Puritan's Pride at **www.puritan.com.**

3. Valerian: Valerian is especially popular with herbalists and anxiety sufferers alike, because it reduces anxiety as well as muscle tension.

The unique substances, which include valerenic acid and valerenon, not only work alone, but they enhance the effects of other substances. This means that valerian should not be taken with sleeping pills, or anxiety medication. You can buy Nature's Answer Valerian Root in 500 mg doses at **www.iherb.com.**

4. Exercise: Studies have shown that physical exercise increases the neurotransmitter dopamine and is a powerful solution to anxiety, as well as depression and other related problems. If you don't already exercise, you should start slowly by doing something you enjoy.

Take a 30-minute morning stroll every day, or spend time daily working in the garden. In addition to getting some exercise, this sun exposure will help regulate your hormone levels, which can go a long way toward relieving anxiety.

STOP THOSE MIDNIGHT BATHROOM RUNS — BEFORE THEY WRECK YOUR SLEEP

To get a good night's sleep, you need your whole body to cooperate — and that goes double for your bladder.

But as we get older, lots of us guys learn that keeping our bladders in line is easier said than done.

Many guys are getting up five or six times… or more… a night for bathroom runs. And that can make getting the sleep you need next to impossible.

I'm sure you've heard before that the problem is probably your prostate. It's common for a man's prostate to enlarge with age — and a swollen prostate can put pressure on your bladder or keep your bladder from fully emptying.

The next thing you know, you're up every hour sprinting for the toilet.

That's no way to live… and the good news is that you don't have to live that way anymore. Because I'm about to introduce you to…

The African secret for TOTAL bladder control

Yes, believe it or not, there's a powerful natural substance that can whip both your bladder and your prostate back into shape in just a few weeks' time.

That means fewer bathroom runs — and much better sleep — for you.

It's called pygeum, and it comes from a cherry tree that grows in the mountainous regions throughout Africa.

And it's been used by African tribespeople for centuries to relieve bladder problems. Those same tribal people even introduced it to early African explorers, who brought pygeum back to Europe with them.

In fact, if you visit a doctor in Europe for a swollen prostate, there's a good chance you'll end up leaving with pygeum instead of some heavy-duty Big Pharma drug like Proscar.

It's actually approved as a treatment for benign prostatic hyperplasia in Germany, France, and Italy.

But because of the way that the billion-dollar drug companies control medicine in America, many guys (and their doctors) have never heard a word about this amazing prostate treatment.

And that's a real shame, because the research behind pygeum is nothing short of remarkable.

Even the University of Michigan Health System calls it, "Safe and effective for men with mild to moderate BPH." (Too bad more mainstream doctors don't check out their website).

In a study out of Europe, 85 men with BPH were took 50 mg of pygeum twice a day for two months.

And TWO MONTHS was all it took for these guys to experience a whopping 40 percent reduction in their prostate symptoms.

But here's the best part...

They were getting up 32 percent LESS at night to pee!

What would one-third fewer bathroom trips mean for your sleep — and your health?

And, trust me, pygeum isn't a one-trick pony. It's backed by decades of research and clinical trials.

In another study, men with BPH took 100 mg of pygeum or placebo daily for the same two months.

And the results were just as impressive. I'm talking about nearly one-third fewer trips to the toilet at night, and about 25 percent less bladder volume left over after they peed.

They were emptying their bladders more completely... and, more importantly, less frequently.

A staggering 66 percent of the men on pygeum reported improvements. Let's see Big Pharma compete with that.

So what's pygeum's secret? It contains compounds called pentacyclic triterpenoids, which have a diuretic effect that can help empty your bladder. And pygeum is also chock-full of phytosterols, which help keep inflammation in check.

Pygeum has the potential to be truly life-changing for guys who are getting up throughout the night to pee.

And while you'll probably never hear about it from mainstream doctors, this is one case where you can take matters into your own hands.

In both of the studies I cited, the dose of pygeum used was 100 mg a day (either as one dose or two 50 mg doses).

And you can find that exact amount in herbal supplements on the market.

You can buy Piping Rock Ultra Standardized Pygeum in 100 mg capsules at **www.pipingrock.com.**

You'll also often find pygeum combined with other prostate-healthy ingredients like saw palmetto and beta sitosterol in multi-ingredient formulas.

CHAPTER TEN

LIVE LONGER (& LOOK YOUNGER) WITH THESE UNDERGROUND BREAKTHROUGHS

AMAZING "CRYSTAL BALL TEST" PREDICTS HOW LONG YOU'LL LIVE

I've been practicing medicine for 35 years.

And if there's one thing we docs love to do, it's throw around numbers.

I'm sure you've noticed, right?

We'll talk about your systolic blood pressure, your triglyceride count, or your Hb1Ac... and somehow you're supposed to put this all together and figure out what kind of health you're in.

It's no wonder so many patients leave their doctors' offices with their heads swimming!

But, believe it or not, there's a simple test you can do at home, that will give you the real scoop on your health.

In fact, it can actually predict how likely you are to die in the next six years.

That's a scary concept, I know.

But the best part of this test is that it can spot serious health problems years before they may show up on mainstream tests... and it can give you an important window to turn your health around.

The Major Health Risk Most Doctors Ignore

Before I explain how to perform this life-saving test at home, it's important to understand exactly what it's measuring — and why it's important.

Because I can practically guarantee this is something your doctor has never discussed with you before.

What we're going to assess is something called "functional movement" — and it goes all the way back to our caveman days.

For a moment, place yourself in the shoes (or, more accurately, the bare feet) of these earliest humans.

There were no cars, trains, planes or boats. You had to walk, run, crawl, or even swim to get where you needed to go.

There were no grocery stores or restaurants, so you had to chase down, dig up, and carry what you wanted to eat.

Because there was no plumbing, if you wanted water, you had to get down to ground level and drink from the surface of a creek or pond, or, scoop it into a container and carry it.

Basically, we had to support own bodies, or we were a-goner. We developed strong hips, and the ability to squat, throw, run, climb, swim and lift heavy objects. This sculpted everything from our muscles, joints, and tendons to our nervous system and internal organs.

That's right... this type of everyday activity, called functional movement, actually stimulates receptors in our bodies that affect our organs and how our genes express themselves. And, as more and more research proves, that all adds up to how long you live.

So what happens if you spend all day letting our modern conveniences do everything for you, without much functional movement?

The result will be hip and knee replacements, blown

discs, and also degenerative diseases like diabetes, cognitive decline, or even cancer.

The best way to extend your life is to incorporate more functional movement into your daily routine, like lifting, walking, squatting, or crawling. In other words, to have the health and the long life you deserve, you need to compensate for all the ways that modern conveniences are screwing us up.

Fortunately, there's a simple, do-it-yourself test that can tell you what kind of functional movement ability you have… and what you may have lost over the years.

Science has actually proven that this test is like a crystal ball that can predict your risk of dying in the next six years.

Even if you think you're in pretty good shape, the results of this test may surprise you. But the good news is that you'll be getting this information while you still have time to make some important changes.

The Crystal Ball Test For Living Longer

An easy way to measure your ability to perform functional movement is the Sitting-Rising-Test (SRT).

The test involves a score of 0–5 for each movement (sitting and rising), with a combined 10 being the highest score that is awarded for those who can sit and rise from the floor without any assistance from their hands or knees.

While appearing simple, it gauges several important factors, including your muscle strength, flexibility, balance and motor coordination, all of which are important to your overall health.

To perform the test, sit down on the floor and then get up, using as little assistance from your hands, knees or other body parts as possible. For each body part that you use for support, you'll lose one point from the possible top score of 10.

As an example, if you put one hand on the floor for support

to sit down, then use a knee and a hand to help you get up, you would lose three points for a combined score of 7.

If you lose your balance, then a half-point is deducted.

Research shows your SRT score strongly correlates with your risk of death within the next six years.

But the good news? For each one-point increase in SRT score, study subjects gained a 21 percent improvement in survival. That sounds pretty good, right?

OK, so take a moment to perform the test and give yourself a score. Once you have your number, here's what the research says:

- Those who scored 0–3 were 6.5 times more likely to die during the six-year-long study than those who scored 8–10.
- Those who scored 3.5–5.5 were 3.8 times more likely to die within the next six years.
- Those who scored 6–7.5 were 1.8 times more likely to die within the next six years.

Need to Boost Your Score? Here's How

Now, I know, the results of this test can be discouraging for some people. I've had these conversations with more patients than I can count.

One thing I hear a lot is that we've evolved past these early cavemen and learned to adapt to our environment.

Well, the people who have completely adapted to our modern environment, and whose spines perfectly fit their recliners, won't look that great. They won't be making the cover of *Men's Health* magazine, or the swimsuit edition of *Sports Illustrated*. And, research shows, they won't live that long, either.

So how do you improve your SRT score? Well, the first step, as I said, is to try to compensate for all the modern conveniences we take too much advantage of.

Take that short talk to the post office, instead of using your car. Carry your own bags out of the grocery store, instead of relying on the clerk. If you have a regular exercise routine, focus on time of day. Believe it or not, that matters a lot.

Many people are early morning exercisers, because they want to get it out of the way. Our bodies, however, tend to respond better with forceful movements in the late afternoon.

If you work out hard before sun exposure, there is more damage to the structural protein in our joints, collagen.

This gets a little scientific, but collagen is actually unzipped from its structure in the early morning by the hormone cortisol and then is re-zipped by the energy from daily sun exposure.

That is why it's good to get some sun exposure in the morning, but to exercise in the late afternoon if you can. That strengthens your collagen and protects it from injury and degradation. Also, I would recommend consulting with a certified Functional Movement Specialist or a certified MovNat trainer. This expert can evaluate your movement patterns and prescribe corrective exercises to improve your functional movement abilities.

You can find a Functional Movement Specialist near you at **www.functionalmovement.com** (just click "Find Certified Members"). For a MovNat trainer, go to **www.movnat.com/find-a-trainer/**.

Bonus Content! Is That Gym Membership Really Helping You?

There are lots of people who don't want to think about functional movement, because they're convinced that they're already in good shape.

They all say the same thing… or something close to it.

They'll talk about how they're walking six miles on the treadmill, four times a week.

Well, those folks may be good at walking on a treadmill, but I don't think this activity will help their health that much. That even goes for athletes.

The repetitive movement doesn't give us the variety that we need to develop a healthy body. I would tell a person that walking on the treadmill indoors is foreign to the musculoskeletal system and senses. It's an abnormal surface and there are abnormal neurological inputs.

After all, where in nature could you walk six miles on a rubberized, moving surface with no stimuli other than the fake, indoor light bombarding your eyes?

The bottom line is that you need to envision what a primitive human had to do in a day to survive and then duplicate it, if you want to have the health that you were designed to have.

Keep your exercise practical and outdoors as much as possible. You'll improve your health, strengthen muscles you didn't even know you had, and maybe save a bundle on gym memberships.

ADD YEARS TO YOUR LIFE WITH THIS FORBIDDEN BEVERAGE

I can't tell you how many patients I've treated over the years who were told to give up coffee by some well-meaning doctor.

I can't imagine starting the day without the smell of fresh-brewed coffee.

And I don't want you to imagine it either. Because coffee is yet another thing that the mainstream has been wrong about for years.

Coffee isn't bad for your health. In fact…

This wonder beverage could literally add years to your life!

The science proves it. A massive study from the journal *Circulation,* published in 2015, actually looked at doctors and nurses who drank coffee (and who didn't).

When they factored out smokers (can you believe there are doctors and nurses who smoke?), researchers found that a regular coffee habit decreases your chances of dying by an impressive 15 percent.

And the more coffee these folks drank, the greater the benefit.

Put in terms of years, that means a person could theoretically gain years of life if they were expected to reach the usual lifespan of an American.

You heard that right — drinking coffee could possibly add years to your life versus not drinking it at all.

The most benefit seems to come from about 3–5 cups a day, and here's the best part.

It doesn't matter if the coffee is caffeinated or decaf. So even if you have trouble handling caffeine, you can still get the benefits of coffee.

Which diseases does coffee seem to prevent the most?

Researchers saw significant reductions in mortality associated with cardiovascular disease, neurological disease and suicide.

But, of course, we know that the benefits of coffee don't end there.

Previous studies show that compounds in coffee improve blood sugar and reduce the risk of diabetes.

This would go hand-in-hand with reducing the risk of cardiovascular disease because diabetes is such a big risk factor for that.

Other studies have shown that coffee reduces the risk of Parkinson's disease, so it would make sense that coffee lowers neurological disease death rates.

Coffee's secret, as I mentioned, is not the caffeine. Your morning cup of joe is actually loaded with antioxidants that help fight damaging free radicals, and coffee also reduces inflammation (a key risk factor for many diseases).

So if you swore off coffee long ago, it may be time to start brewing it up again. Your health will be better for it.

SUSANNAH'S SECRETS TO LIVING TO 116 (YOU'RE GOING TO LOVE THEM)

And as long as we're talking about "forbidden" treats… let me tell you a story about Susannah, from Brooklyn, NY.

Susannah died in 2016, just a couple of months before she turned 117. She was in the Guinness World Records at the time as the oldest living human.

Why do I bring her up?

We should be looking at people with great longevity to see if there is anything in their lifestyles that might have contributed to their outstanding health.

And there's plenty you can learn from Susannah to live the long and healthy life you deserve.

Susannah was born in 1899 in Alabama, and she worked picking crops on a farm.

That actually comes with some health advantages.

I'm talking about adequate sun exposure and grounding to the earth. Susannah had lots of opportunity to power up her vitamin D synthesis, for sulfation of cholesterol, and for stimulation of the photopigments in the retina that affect our hormone balance.

Someone asked Susannah what her secret was for a long life. She answered bacon and eggs in the morning and lots of sleep.

She also mentioned close social and family connections.

I know there's a big movement by some medical practitioners pushing for a plant-based diet, but here we have an example of a woman eating bacon and eggs every day of her life and living longer than anyone else.

Mainstream nutrition and medicine said forever that saturated fats are bad and one of the causes of cancer and coronary disease, which are among the leading causes of death in America.

I know things are slowly changing — for the better in my opinion. In fact, the American Council on Nutrition, which is the group that oversees registered dietitians, has recently revised their nutritional recommendations stating that they no longer recommend worrying about saturated fat or cholesterol in the diet.

Now that is a big change — but Susannah was onto it decades ago.

Like most animal foods, bacon contains protein, vitamins and minerals and is a particularly good source of choline and sulfur which tend to be low in a processed food or vegan diet.

Eggs are one of the richest sources of choline in the diet. Saturated fats are a clean source of energy and energy drives life.

Of course, there are a couple of caveats here. Please avoid the man-made saturated fats, like trans fats and highly processed vegetable oils.

Avoid bacon from industrial farms where the animals have poor living conditions and tend to be unhealthy. Natural and local is the way I like to go.

I would also recommend not cooking the bacon at high

temperature, as this can create cancer-causing compounds.

And it's not just Susannah who thrived by enjoying some crispy slices of bacon daily.

Gertrude Barnes, who lived to 115 years and was also the world's oldest living person at one time, lived on a diet of regular bacon.

Edna Parker lived to be 115 as well with a diet dominated by eggs, bacon and fried chicken.

We are talking about the elite of the elite here. The oldest people on the planet.

They might be telling us something.

HERE'S EXACTLY HOW MUCH VITAMIN D I RECOMMEND

It seems like everyone is on the vitamin D bandwagon today — and that includes me.

Vitamin D is critical to so many biological processes, and having enough is key to warding off many of the degenerative diseases we face as we age,

For years, I've been personally trying to get more sun exposure and eat more foods that contain vitamin D.

In my patients, I advise the same.

Also, after measuring vitamin D levels in the blood, in the past I would have patients taking 5,000 IU of vitamin D3 supplements daily. I changed this advice when most of the clinical trials on giving vitamin D supplements did not shown significant health benefits. So now I advise more sun if vitamin D is low.

And what kinds of benefits can you expect from higher vitamin D levels? I saw an article in *Life Extension* magazine that summarized some of the vitamin D research in a table.

If you're low in vitamin D, here's how much you are increasing your risk of the following diseases:

- **Multiple Sclerosis:** 61% increase
- **Psoriasis:** 189% increase
- **Bladder Cancer:** 83% increase overall;
  494% for invasive tumors
- **Breast Cancer:** 150% increase
- **Thyroid Cancer:** 100% increase
- **Cognitive Decline:** 41%–60% increase
- **Risk of Heart Attack:** 38%–192% increase
- **Alzheimer's:** 2,000% increase
- **Respiratory Infection:** 36% increase
- **Diabetes:** 91% increase for insulin resistance,
  38%–106% for type 2 diabetes
- **Diabetes** (risk of progression from normal
  to high blood sugar): 77% increase
- **Stroke:** 22%–64% increase

I suspect there's still much we're learning about vitamin D. As an example, sardines are a great source of D along with the other oily fish. And we know that ultraviolet light catalyzes the formation of vitamin D, but this light doesn't penetrate water well.

So the question is, how do the fish get it? A recent study shows that both phytoplankton and zooplankton form vitamin D. And so does grass.

That's why taking grazing animals off their natural food (and loading them up with cheap feed, as many factory farms do) may reduce the health value of animal foods.

If you work indoors and eat processed food, take 5,000 IU of supplemental vitamin a day for chance to get the wide array of health benefits seen in the studies.

USE THIS CHEMICAL REACTION TO SLOW AGING TO A CRAWL

It seems like when it comes to aging science, methylation is the one process that nobody is talking about.

But if you want to be one of those people who looks 20 years younger than you are… if you want to still be hitting the golf links or dance floor in your 70s or 80s… methylation is something you need to know about and master.

This can get a little complicated and scientific. But hang with me — it'll be worth it.

Methylation is a chemical reaction where a methyl group (which is a carbon atom attached to 3 hydrogen atoms) binds to another molecule.

And here's why that's important. Methylation is one of the factors that controls how our DNA and genes are expressed… and it can slow the negative expression of genes.

In other words, *it can help slow aging to a crawl.*

Methylation determines your rate of glutathione synthesis. Glutathione is critical for detoxification and antioxidant function (so it keeps us healthy), and methylation also helps our immune systems fight off infections.

Methylation even lowers levels of homocysteine, which can prevent heart attacks and strokes. A study reported in *JAMA* showed 3.4 times more strokes and heart attacks in people with high homocysteine versus those with low levels.

Methylation produces S-adenosylmethionine (SAMe), which may have potent anti-aging effects, and has been shown to alleviate depression, improve Alzheimer's and Parkinson's disease patients, help arthritis, and protect against alcohol-induced liver injury.

Protecting DNA, as methylation does, may reduce the risk of genetically induced cancers, too.

So by enhancing methylation, we may be able to improve health and slow premature, and maybe even normal, aging.

And there are plenty of things you can do to enhance methylation in your body.

One of the easiest ways is by eating plenty of vegetables.

You can also enhance methylation by supplementation with nutrients like folate, vitamin B12, vitamin B6, choline and most importantly, trimethylglycine (TMG).

Conventional medical journals such as *JAMA* have recommended vitamin supplements such as folic acid as safe methods of lowering homocysteine.

A more effective nutrient to lower homocysteine is TMG. TMG converts homocysteine into methionine and, in the process, produces SAMe.

SAMe is prescribed as a drug in Europe and is available here in the United States, but is fairly expensive. TMG is inexpensive and is readily available as a dietary supplement.

TMG and SAMe both facilitate youthful methylation metabolism. Enhancing methylation not only protects against many diseases, but may make your biochemistry younger and you may feel younger.

Many people feel better when supplementing with TMG because of the beneficial effects of elevated SAMe.

Improving methylation will help your immune system and detoxification, too.

But, and this is a big but, if you have infections or loads of toxins, you might feel worse before you feel better. That's common with any detoxification process.

I recommend supplementing TMG with the help of a nutritional coach or doctor who has vast experience.

A coach can warn you and give you the support you need to get through the period where you may feel worse — before you get better.

THE ANTI-AGING SUPERFOOD MOST AMERICANS DON'T KNOW ABOUT

We all know that we need to get more healthy fats and nutrients into our diets… especially if we want to slow aging and prevent disease.

There's one food that's a nutritional powerhouse and that I regularly eat and recommend to my patients.

And most of them have never heard of it.

This food is called ghee or clarified butter.

In Ayurvedic healing, ghee is regularly used to improve digestion, one of the most pressing needs of our population.

It's also known to slow the aging process and improve immunity, and is thought to increase intelligence and memory. Ghee even has properties that aid in detoxification.

Ghee is different from butter in that the moisture, proteins and sugars are removed through the clarification process. This makes ghee a pure fat, which doesn't need to be refrigerated.

It's made by boiling butter for an hour and a half, or longer, to remove the moisture and cause the precipitation of the proteins and sugars contained in butter.

One advantage of ghee over butter is that it has a much higher smoke point, so it has much more versatility in cooking. It also contains more medium chain triglycerides than butter, which have been shown to have metabolism benefits.

Ghee would also be better for anyone with an allergy to milk or lactose intolerance because the casein and lactose are removed.

Better still, ghee contains vitamin A, vitamin K2 and conjugated linoleic acid (CLA). The average person doesn't get enough of these important nutrients in their diet, so ghee is a great food to add to your menu.

K2 is important for our arteries and bones. CLA improves our metabolism and helps with weight loss and preventing diabetes. Vitamin A is a powerful antioxidant and is critical for many physiologic functions in the body, including our vision.

The problem today with many of the foods that we consume is the industrialization of the food supply, and this certainly applies to the processing of dairy products.

I prefer my ghee to be made from raw milk and from cows eating grass.

If milk is pasteurized and homogenized, it's not the same as natural milk. I recommend that the butter, from which ghee is made, is churned in a traditional fashion. The problem is most butter today, even organic butter, is made with an extrusion processes instead of churning.

So the ideal way of getting ghee is to make it yourself from raw milk (you can easily find recipes online).

If that's not possible, more grocery stores are starting to carry it, and if you have an Indian grocery store nearby, you're sure to find it.

CAN FASTING KEEP YOU YOUNG? ONLY IF YOU DO IT RIGHT

It seems like every diet and detox program out there today recommends fasting.

They want you to practically starve yourself, all in the name of keeping you healthy.

Well, that doesn't sound like a whole lot of fun for me — and, I'll tell you, it's an awfully tough sell with my patients.

But the fact is, there is a type of fasting that can improve your health and even help you age better. And, unlike a lot of the other programs out there, my fasting protocol won't leave you in a constant state of misery.

It all starts with a cellular process called autophagy.

This is where our cells recycle debris that tends to build up — and it's incredibly healthy.

Many times this debris is from dysfunctional organelles like the mitochondria. The mitochondria are the organelles that produce energy and they can commonly malfunction and become broken, creating health problems.

It's like the cell is saying, "Hey, we need to take out the trash or die a cluttered death."

Autophagy is part of our natural defense system and is one of the major ways that our cells fight invaders such as viruses, bacteria and parasites.

Certain infectious diseases have learned to disable autophagy. Organisms that can do this include herpes simplex virus 1, cytomegalovirus and the Epstein-Barr virus, which all can become chronic infections.

Autophagy also can defend against malfunctioning cells such as precancerous or cancerous cells. Research has shown that when our autophagy system is broken, our health dramatically spirals downward.

So you want to encourage autophagy — and that starts with LIMITED fasting.

Autophagy is turned on when the cell is deprived of nutrients, such as after a fast. This tends to happen after about 12 hours of fasting.

So if you're one of those people who snack all day, you're going to have a hard time encouraging autophagy.

One easy way to stimulate autophagy is to skip a meal, like breakfast. You'll hit your 12 hours easily enough.

But this is where a lot of folks in the health industry get it wrong. They figure that if a 12-hour fast is good, a three-day fast must be better.

Not true. Studies show a longer fast does not increase autophagy any more than the shorter fast.

Long-term fasting has the negative aspect of actually inhibiting autophagy once eating has resumed. So until this process is better understood, I recommend considering skipping breakfast several times a week to enhance autophagy.

What I do is eat my evening meal, have no snacks in the evening, and then skip breakfast and instead break the fast at lunch the next day. This works like a charm.

Before you do this, however, I always recommend

listening to your body. If you have food cravings, light-headedness or other symptoms, you should probably eat.

You might want to start with a 12 hour fast and try to build it up to the 16 hour fast that I do. But always pay attention to how you're feeling.

WHEN IT COMES TO THESE DNA STRANDS, SIZE MATTERS

Would you believe that inside your cells are strands of DNA material that can practically predict your future?

They determine how long you'll live... how healthy you'll be... and your chances of coming down with dozens of degenerative diseases.

But most people have never had this DNA tested — and are never told by their doctors that a test is available.

I'll tell you all about this test (and how you can get it in a moment). But first let me explain more about this remarkable collection of DNA called telomeres.

Telomeres are the DNA at the end of our chromosomes — and they are not actually part of the genetic code.

Instead, they act to protect the ends of the chromosomes and prevent them from unraveling. Think of them like caps on the ends of shoelaces.

One study showed that telomeres tend to shorten each time the cell replicates and that telomere length correlates with cellular aging.

So, in a nutshell...

**Keep your telomeres long and you'll age better —
simple as that.**

Scientists have observed that when telomeres are shorter, disease and death may be near. One study with a 6.1 year follow-up showed a significant increase in death from infectious diseases with people who had shorter telomeres.

So it's a sign of our immune systems slowing down and becoming less functional.

I test telomere length often in my patients, along with other biomarkers of aging such as hormone levels, inflammation, and blood chemistry. I also often recommend hair mineral analysis.

The telomere test is particularly important for those people who think that their health is in good shape, but want to be sure.

I think of the case of my friend who did endurance exercise on a regular basis and had a great diet. One day, while riding his bike, he had a heart attack and died at the age of 50.

What would his telomere test have told us? I don't know for sure but chances are his telomeres would've been much shorter than the average for his age.

And when I find short telomeres in my patients, then we know we must make some changes and dig deeper.

It's a common problem with people who do a lot of exercise and assume it will keep them healthy. In general, exercise is a healthy activity — but when it's done on top of other bad habits, like ignoring nutrition, toxins, poor sleep, electromagnetic field exposures and stress, it can actually accelerate the aging process.

I find that these people can look good but often have short telomeres.

Now on the other hand if someone is morbidly obese, has type II diabetes, sleep apnea and peripheral neuropathy, the telomere test might not be so important because you already know the horse has left the barn, and you have more immediate health problems you need to address.

The actual lab results of the telomere test are printed out on a graph that shows the average telomere length plotted against age. The goal is to have long telomeres for your age.

The next question might be, "Can I lengthen my telomeres?"

A prospective study of women reported in the *American Journal of Clinical Nutrition* in 2009 showed that taking a multivitamin increased telomere length by 5 percent versus women that were not taking one.

Other studies have shown a correlation between telomere length and vitamin D status, nutrition, the omega-3 fatty acids EPA and DHA, and calorie restriction in mice.

So there are certainly some steps you can take to preserve and even lengthen your telomeres. But the first step is so get your telomeres measured.

The test is available from SpectraCell Laboratories for a retail price of around $300 and can be ordered by your doctor.

12 DAYS TO A HEALTHIER (AND LONGER) LIFE

We're all creatures of habit — for better or worse.

If you're in the habit of watching 6 hours of TV a day and laying around on the couch, you're in a cycle that will eventually undermine your health.

But if you start positive, healthy habits, you can prevent — and even reverse — many of the degenerative diseases we associate with aging.

These are the types of habits I try to encourage in my patients. And it starts with a 12-day challenge.

I want you to spend the next 12 days trying to incorporate each of these habits into your daily routine.

Just add one a day.

You'll find that each of these habits help you produce more cellular energy, detoxify your body, burn fat, and build up your stores of critical nutrients.

In short, they're going to make you feel younger and better than you have in years. My own patients are living proof.

Day 1: Begin drinking pure spring water. Glass containers are best but plastic containers are acceptable. If you live near a spring, you can collect your own water and you may be able to find a spring at **findaspring.com.** It is very important to avoid fluoridated water, which is toxic to our cells.

Day 2: Get up early and face the sun as it rises over the horizon. You look in the direction of the sun with no glasses, contacts or windows to obstruct your view.

This can be done anywhere from 1 to 20 minutes and you do not look directly at the sun but off to the side. The simple act will set the circadian clock in the suprachiasmatic nucleus of the brain, which is critical for optimal health.

Day 3: Pick out a time later in the morning when UVA light is present in the sunlight. This will vary with latitude and season, but is generally around 9 AM.

Again, with the eyes uncovered by contacts, glasses or windows, you face the sun and allow the UV light to enter the retina area where it activates the creation of dopamine and melatonin in the retina. This can be done anywhere from 5 to 20 minutes.

Start with shorter times and gradually increase as tolerated. Check with your doctor if you have eye conditions.

Day 4: Begin UVB sun exposure. The time of UVB will vary depending on latitude. The D Minder app (available in all major app stores) will tell you what hours UVB is present.

Preferably in the morning, around 10 AM in the summer months, start with 5 to 60 minutes. The longer times are needed based on how much skin is exposed, season, latitude and your starting skin color. The D Minder takes these variables into account.

Day 5: Begin a daily dose of nature. This could be a walk in a park or natural area. It is important to have quiet time in nature where you're out, being exposed to the sun. It's good to be grounded if possible (bare foot or touching the ground with your skin).

Day 6: Begin eliminating your exposure to artificial light (like the kinds we get from electronic devices and modern light bulbs) after the sun goes down. Artificial light is high in the blue spectrums that lower melatonin levels. That has multiple negative effects on our health, including disrupting sleep.

Blue light in our modern lights also disturbs the circadian rhythm which is critical for optimal health. Options are blue blocking glasses (I use Uvex, which you can buy at **www.amazon.com**), screen covers, turning lights off, and replacing CFLs and LEDs with Amber-colored lights.

Day 7: Begin grounding or earthing. This is where you go barefoot or place other body parts onto non-electrified ground. This can be concrete, dirt, grass, beach, rock, a body of water or another natural surface.

This will actually transfer electrons from the Earth that your body's cells can use for energy. The minimum amount of time required is thought to be about 20 minutes. This should be the minimum amount of time spent on grounding each day.

Day 8: Begin face dunking (I describe this more in my weight-loss chapter). This is where you take a bowl or sink of ice water, hold your breath and dunk your face in the water, keeping it in as long as you can. Monitor the times.

This stimulates the production of healthy brown fat.

Do this for a total of 2 to 3 minutes per day. See if you can increase the time that you can hold your breath and you'll quickly notice how the discomfort decreases each day and the ability to hold your breath improves. Cold showers are another option.

Day 9: Eat a low-mercury source of seafood (and aim to do this at least three days a week). Sardines, wild caught salmon, and shellfish are optimal. All seafood is acceptable.

Seafood is necessary to obtain adequate DHA, which is incorporated into the cell membranes and allows the transmission of energy for optimal cellular functioning and energy production.

Day 10: Begin to incorporate natural movement. Humans had millions of years where they performed certain movements that were required for survival.

Movement affects the positive, healthy expression of our genetic code.

If you think of a primitive human as having to walk and move to find and gather food, carry water, build a shelter, migrate, chase down prey or run from danger, etc., you can see that we're designed to move in ways that our modern lives have extinguished.

Begin by doing some simple natural movements like walking barefoot on an uneven surface, squatting, pulling yourself up with your arms, and other activities you might envision a primitive human doing.

If we get away from natural movements, it will result in the abnormal expression of our genes, which has led to the current widespread disease and dysfunction of our musculoskeletal and nervous systems.

Driving somewhere? Walk instead. Instead of putting your groceries in a cart, carry them. If you want to get a good look at a flower on the side of the trail, or look a small child in the eye, squat down and get real close.

Incorporate these activities in baby steps. Some people will have physical limitations that will make some of these positions or movements impossible. Be creative and have fun.

Day 11: Begin a time for meditation each day. Sit or lie in a quiet place where you're unlikely to be disturbed. It's usually best if you close your eyes.

Take some deep breaths were you slowly fill the chest and the abdomen with air and then breathe out completely. Try to empty your mind of all thoughts and focus on your breathing.

You may want to envision breathing light into your chest that spreads into your body. With the light entering the body, try to feel that energy, which may be a tingling or a weightless sensation.

It's often easier first to feel the tingling in the hands. Focus on the feeling.

Thoughts may arise. If a thought comes into your mind, acknowledge what it is but don't judge it or deal with it.

Try to draw your attention back to the feeling of energy in your body or your hands. However many times it takes, be patient and draw your attention back to your hands and on the feeling of your internal energy.

You can do this for 10 to 15 minutes once or twice a day. As you practice, you will become more skilled at identifying the feeling of energy that is contained within your body and increase your ability to keep your focus on the present moment.

Day 12: You begin to reduce non-native electromagnetic field exposure. This could be something as simple as frequently turning off your cell phone, keeping it far from your body, or placing it in airplane mode.

It's especially important not to have wireless devices or electronic devices close to where you sleep. You can often disconnect Wi-Fi at night.

Electrical currents also create electric and magnetic fields that have an impact on cellular function.

It's best to sleep at least 6 feet away from any type of electrical cord or electronic device.

There are other possible sources of electromagnetic pollution such as cell phone towers, microwave ovens, smart meters and many energy-saving appliances. The best way to fully mitigate your environment is to have it tested for radio-frequency fields, electric fields, magnetic fields and dirty electricity.

CHAPTER ELEVEN

10 MORE LIFE-CHANGING BONUS TIPS

HERE'S EXACTLY HOW MUCH WATER YOU SHOULD BE DRINKING

Ask the mainstream medical establishment how much water you need every day, and you get the same pat answer.

They want you drinking 8 glasses.

Not exactly helpful, is it? I mean, how big is a glass? And what type of water? And are you really recommending the same water intake for a 300-pound man as a 100-pound woman?

This is another example where the medical system has over-simplified something that is very important, and left everyone confused.

There's no doubt that water is vital to countless biological and chemical processes that are happening in our bodies all the time.

We have more molecules of water in our bodies than anything else. That's why you hear people say we're made out of water.

In a way, we are.

Water basically helps charge and power our cells. Our brains are bathed in cerebral spinal fluid which over 99 percent water and this allows our quantum computer (brain) to do the amazing things it can do.

So how much water should you be drinking to stay healthy

— and is there a certain type of water that's best?

The amount of water you need depends on your size and other factors such as temperature and humidity.

As a target for water intake, I generally recommend that a person drink one half their body weight in pounds in ounces of water. So for a 150-pound person a ballpark figure would be 75 ounces of water per day.

This is something you may need to work up to. But if you make water your primary beverage, it's very doable.

And I don't recommend getting water from your tap.

Tap water contains toxins and drug residues, and is usually treated with chemicals.

Some municipalities fluoridate water which is actually toxic to our cells. The mass-fluoridation of our water supply has been a health tragedy that our government still refuses to recognize.

And the evidence that there are any significant dental benefits is shaky at best, believe me.

I recommend you drink spring water, when possible.

If you know of or have access to a spring that is good.

But you can buy it in the store or have it delivered to your home.

I prefer glass containers to limit toxins from the container.

Findaspring.com is a website that lists many springs and in the comments section people might report any testing that has been done on the water. It's a great resource.

If spring water isn't an option for you, I'd recommend investing in a quality water filter.

Look for something that removes fluoride and toxins from the water.

Many water filters will have been tested and rated by laboratories like NSF. Look for those labels and third-party testing that validates that the filter can do what it promises to do.

DON'T LET THIS "WONDER DRUG" STEAL YOUR EYESIGHT

I've spent most of my career busting mainstream medical myths.

And today I want to put the aspirin-a-day nonsense to bed once and for all. There's a ton of research on what this over-the-counter painkiller will do to people, especially seniors — and most of it is bad.

Here's the latest: Take a daily aspirin, and you more than DOUBLE the risk of losing your vision, possibly permanently and completely, to the "wet" form of late-stage macular degeneration, according to a study in the *Archives of Internal Medicine*.

Age-related macular degeneration is **the leading cause of blindness among people over the age of 55.**

The researchers found that the relationship was "dose-dependent" — meaning, the more aspirin you take regularly, the higher the risk of macular degeneration.

Suddenly that daily aspirin isn't sounding so good, right?

And this research is no fluke, either.

It actually confirmed a previous study in the journal *Ophthalmology* that showed EXACTLY the same results: People who take aspirin twice a day have a doubled risk of advanced age-related macular degeneration, compared with people who don't regularly take aspirin.

But it gets worse. In addition to vision loss, studies have linked daily aspirin use to hearing loss, tinnitus, sexual dysfunction and more. It also dramatically boosts your odds of serious internal bleeding.

Now, of course, we're all bombarded with those commercials promising that aspirin can prevent heart attacks, right? Well, not so fast.

A massive analysis in the *American Journal of Cardiology* found that aspirin had NO significant effect in primary prevention for coronary artery disease, strokes, heart-related deaths, or even for overall mortality.

That's right — when used for prevention, it saved NO lives.

How can so many doctors continue the aspirin-a-day mantra?

It has to do with risk vs. benefit. And in all the studies I've seen, the risk/benefit is barely neck and neck — in other words, the risk is about the same as the benefit. For those people who are at high risk for a heart attack or stroke, it might be worth the risk.

For everyone else, it's not.

Aspirin has its place — and that is during an actual heart attack.

Heck, I'd even take one if I was having crushing chest pain.

But for prevention, NO WAY.

Rather than relying on a shortcut that deceives you into thinking you're doing something worthwhile, do what you KNOW is worthwhile.

Eat a natural, nutrient-dense diet with superfoods and raw foods. Use your body for physical work on a daily basis. I guarantee there are more benefits and less risks going this route.

And natural supplements like CoQ10 are great for giving your aging heart an energy boost (I even take it myself).

But whatever you do, don't let anyone sweet-talk you into a daily aspirin for preventing a heart attack.

The only thing you may end up preventing is good health.

USE THIS BATHROOM SECRET TO STOP DOZENS OF DISEASES

Listen, I get it — bathroom time is supposed to be private time.

Just the king and queen and his or her throne.

But, hey, I'm a doctor… and there's an uncomfortable conversation we need to have. It involves the way you poop.

Because what if I told you there was a simple way to reduce your risk of heart attack, stroke, appendicitis, bowel and bladder incontinence, hemorrhoids, hiatal hernia, GERD, colon cancer, irritable bowel disease, inflammatory bowel disease, constipation, small intestine bacterial overgrowth, prostate cancer, diverticulitis, pelvic organ prolapse and possibly more?

And all you have to do is start squatting when you move your bowels.

You can look at cultures that squat to poop versus Western cultures that sit on a throne; there tends to a huge discrepancy in the incidence of the above diseases.

They are rare or missing in the squatting-to-poop

cultures and are extremely common and increasing in Western cultures.

Of course primitive humans didn't sit while they were defecating. That came later when the modern toilet became widespread in the 1800s.

Before that, we squatted and did our dirty deed on the ground, in a pot or maybe in a hole. But now we sit as if we were sitting in a chair.

That may seem convenient, but it's doing a number on your health.

Sitting puts our rectum at the wrong angle so it doesn't allow gravity to aid defecation.

Plus, sitting causes kinks in our rectum which further impedes complete evacuation.

On top of all this, when we're sitting, the puborectalis muscle is pulled tight across the rectum which is the main contributor to humans not soiling themselves and thus not needing a diaper.

The puborectalis is a muscle shaped like a sling that goes around our rectums to keep them closed. This sling-muscle automatically releases its grip on the rectum when we're in the full, squatted position.

But when we sit, we end up holding our breath and straining, which causes a lot of the adverse health consequences I've talked about.

Now, I know what you may be thinking — maybe you haven't gotten into a full squat position in 40 years.

OK, I'll cut you some slack. In that case, you should start today increasing the range of motion of your hips, knees, and ankles and eventually, it is likely you will be able to squat again.

Those with hip or knee replacement or severe osteoarthritis might need to make some modifications to a full squat.

In my view, being able to squat has way more benefits

than just the ones I mentioned already. If a person is able to get in a squatting position and stay there, that means you are able to achieve full range of motion of your weight-bearing joints and spine.

This will help prevent the other epidemic diseases of Western cultures like osteoarthritis, osteoporosis, degenerative spine disease, and the chronic pain associated with these conditions.

So here we have a remedy that is simple, doesn't cost much money, and prevents so many diseases that have the potential to make our lives miserable.

If you are able to squat, there is a simple way to convert your toilet into one you can squat on to defecate.

Take 4 standard cinder blocks, 8 x 8 x 18. With the steel brush, brush off the loose pieces. Then I recommend painting the blocks.

Stack the blocks horizontally on each side of the toilet. Cut out a piece of plywood in a U-shape that goes across the front of your toilet and is open in the back. I would paint this as well, just in case one day you miss, it will clean up better.

Then place the wood on top the cinder block and now you have a toilet where you can squat to defecate.

Once you do this little construction job, for under $10 in cost, you can start down the road to prevent or improve any of those conditions I mentioned above.

It's way better than having a bladder sling inserted, hemorrhoidectomy, prostatectomy, colectomy, appendectomy, hernia repair, or countless other procedures.

If it doesn't work for you, you can always take your home-made contraption out of your bathroom. But if you're like most of my patients, you're going to notice that you can poop more easily and completely — and that you just feel better — right away.

DEMAND THIS TREATMENT DURING YOUR NEXT HOSPITAL STAY

A couple of years ago, I had the health scare of my life.

But what I learned could help you or someone you love recover more quickly — and thoroughly — during your next hospital stay (which I hope is a long, long way off).

One day during the summer of 2015, I was at my office on a Saturday… and I was worried.

My son, Gabe, had asked, "What's wrong with you? You're so slow and bumping into things."

I'd been having a headache in the sinus area for three weeks and was thinking I had better schedule an appointment with a neurologist and get my head scanned.

I went into the restroom in the clinic and took a look at my reflection — and I was horrified.

My right eyelid was drooping — and my life flashed before my eyes.

I pictured my wife and kids at the funeral. I pictured myself in the hospital with IVs and a urinary catheter.

Later that day, I was at my son Robbie's college graduation, where I developed weakness in the left side of my body.

And I knew I couldn't wait to see the neurologist — I had to go to the emergency department NOW.

To make a long story short, the CT scan showed that I had bleeding in my head from a previous trauma. That was a great relief to me, but it was still a serious situation and I had to have urgent brain surgery.

It was my stay in the hospital that was my turning point.

The day after my surgery, I was in the intensive care unit connected to IVs, monitors, urinary catheter, oxygen and a tube going inside my head.

When at home, I'm always concerned about my exposure to artificial light and non-native electromagnetic fields.

In that hospital room I was absolutely bombarded, as all hospital patients are.

That's right — we're literally surrounded by the very things that make us sick, and hospitals have nothing in place to address it.

I could tell my energy was critically low and I asked to be placed in natural sunlight.

And then I got that standard hospital answer you may have heard a thousand times: "That's impossible."

After threatening to leave the hospital against medical advice, they finally let me go out in the sun. I swear that sunlight helped in my recovery more than anything the doctors did (after the surgery).

In the ICU I carefully observed my fellow patients, tubes sticking out of their immobile bodies, being bombarded by the artificial light and electromagnetic fields, and being pumped full of all kinds of drugs.

I took a close look at the staff in the hospital — typically overweight and stressed out.

I thought to myself, this is not a place to get healthy.

But because of the system we have, the hospital is where we send the people who are most vulnerable to a bad environment. And it's because of ignorance.

Everyone has believed the lie that the sun is dangerous and yet it's the source of energy for the entire planet. Everyone believes that artificial light and technology are good, but the evidence continues to mount that they have adverse biological effects.

Remember, when you are in the hospital, you are your own best advocate. Demand that you get sunlight every day, as long as it's safe to move you.

This "sunlight treatment" isn't offered as hospitals… it's not even an afterthought. But it could make a huge difference in your recovery.

THE ONLY WAY YOU SHOULD EAT YOUR FRUITS AND VEGGIES

We've been told our entire lives how important fruits and vegetables are for our health.

But the fact is, they're not as healthy as they used to be — and you may not be getting all the vitamins, minerals, and other benefits that you think.

Let me explain.

If you think about it, almost all of our food comes from plants — that's either directly through eating plants, and indirectly, through eating animals that eat plants.

And then of course there is our digestive process that is breaking down these plant-derived foods into the nutrition we need.

But we should go further upstream and ask the question: What did the plants eat? And then we must consider the plant's digestive tract and the assault on it by modern farming methods.

Soil science tells us that plants can't eat or absorb minerals and or other essential nutrients without some help.

I was looking at a website for the North Carolina State

Agriculture Department that was describing soil and the microbes it contains.

It states that a tablespoon of soil can contain up to 50 billion microbes.

OK, I know this is really creepy, but here's a breakdown of the kind of critters contained in soil. There is a table on the website that states 1 g of soil, that's about half of a thimble, contains:

1. Bacteria, number anywhere from 3 million to 500 million organisms.
2. Actinomycetes, which have characteristics of both bacteria and fungi, 1 to 20 million.
3. Fungi, 5,000 to 1 million.
4. Yeast, 1,000 to 1 million.
5. Protozoa, 1,000 to 500,000.
6. Algae 1,000 to 500,000.
7. Nematodes (worm species), 10 to 5,000.

What's amazing is that all of these organisms work in a symbiotic relationship with the plants. Their function is to help release key nutrients, and particularly the minerals in soil, so that plants can absorb them.

In fact, without this process, the plant can't assimilate any minerals. And that means the fruits and vegetables aren't as nutritious as they should be.

If we look at industrial farmland, where over 90 percent of our food is grown, we find that the microbial numbers in the soil are decreased by 85 percent as opposed to an organic farm.

Studies show that an organic farm soil will contain 4 percent to 6 percent of organic material called humus. The commercial farmland has 0 to 1.5 percent humus, which feeds the microbes.

We can easily imagine how this occurs. On the commercial farmland the soil is drenched in herbicides like glyphosate.

Glyphosate is the active ingredient in Roundup and was originally patented as an antibiotic. And then there are the pesticides that also can kill the microbes as well as the chemical fertilizers.

On an industrial farm, there is almost a phobia against letting any kind of weed or other plant grow. In a natural setting, many different plants are growing, including weeds, which add nutrients to the soil.

A couple years ago, a special report to the United Nations found that by switching farming to small-scale family farms, using organic methods, it is possible to double food production in 5 to 10 years.

The problem is that the big corporations have gained control over our legislators. And they want to sell the billions of pounds of chemical fertilizers, herbicides and pesticides that are destroying our planet and the quality of our food.

So change is going to come slowly, if at all. But there's still plenty you can do.

Buy organic fruits and vegetables whenever possible. That way, you'll know your produce was grown in healthy soil, and that it contains the nutrients it should.

Does organic produce cost more? Sure.

But I would argue it's a question of value, not cost. And what's that cheap, mass-produced tomato really worth anyway, if it doesn't contain the critical vitamins, minerals, and other nutrients you need?

THE COMMON DRUG REACTION THAT COULD LAND YOU IN THE ER

We've all heard a bit about anaphylaxis or anaphylactic shock — and it's usually when an allergic child eats a peanut or gets stung by a bee.

And when we go racing for the EpiPen injections.

Anaphylaxis is the result of an allergic reaction that can cause a serious drop in blood pressure and sometimes swelling of the upper respiratory tract that can result in death.

But what is the most common cause of anaphylaxis? It's not peanuts or bees.

A recent study finds that it is most likely to be drugs prescribed by your doctor.

In fact, if you combine all the foods, bites and sting deaths from anaphylaxis, and then TRIPLE that number, you will get to the deaths caused by drug anaphylaxis.

Because there is no registry for anaphylaxis deaths, many times the drugs are never named.

When the drug was named, 40 percent of the time it was an antibiotic.

Another leading cause of drug anaphylaxis was

radiocontrast agents used when doctors are performing CT scans or MRIs with contrast. The other was chemotherapy drugs used to treat cancer.

This should be a warning about the temptation to take an antibiotic for cold.

An antibiotic will have no effect on the virus that's causing your cold. It will not only disrupt the normal flora in your intestine, but it just might cause an anaphylactic reaction as well.

What I do personally when I'm coming down with a cold?

I use an over-the-counter silver solution that I get in the health food store. It's great for treating a cold because not only does silver treat bacterial infections but it also treats viruses.

Drugs have their place, but it is far less than what the typical doctor prescribes. Ask questions and find out about possible alternatives.

READ THIS WARNING BEFORE YOU EAT ANY CHICKEN DISH

Chicken has become a staple of the American diet… and, believe me, I get it. All of my patients eat it, too.

And I understand why — it's an affordable source of protein.

But when you go to the supermarket these days, you notice something awfully unhealthy about modern chickens.

When I look in the poultry case, I see chickens with breasts the size of footballs — and that's not normal.

But what's worse is that when you bite into one of these chicken breasts, it's like biting into a donut. It's pasty and it doesn't have any fibers.

When I get chickens from the local farmer, the chickens breasts have fibers like a muscle would, and the legs are big and strong.

But in the supermarket, birds have absolutely no striations in the meat at all, like it's some kind of mass of cells with no differentiation into a muscle.

It's almost as if you were eating a tumor!

And here's the problem. Big-Agra controls every aspect of the raising of these chickens, which includes feeding them genetically-modified feed laced with growth-promoting additives like antibiotics and hormones.

The chicken farmers get the special, mutant fast-growing chicks from the factory along with the feed.

If you talk to the farmers, they don't even know what's in the feed and they're not allowed to ask because it's all a trade secret.

Awfully suspicious, right?

I found that 40 years ago a broiler, which is what they call a young chicken raised to be eaten by a human being, would be ready for the market in about 84 days.

Today, the broiler is ready in 37 days. How would you like it if your lifespan was 37 days?

The chickens I get from the farmer locally have lived over a year before they're big enough for market.

In the typical factory farm they have 17 birds per square meter, which means that the birds are virtually on top of one another.

And get this — even though they are so young, less than 37 days old, they often develop obesity, heart disease and skeletal deformities because they can't even turn around in the cage because of the overcrowding.

These 37-day-old chickens are like 90-year-old men!

So when you're eating one of those mushy, chicken breasts, you're eating a diseased bird that probably has heart failure.

In the wild, animals won't eat other diseased animals. But we're being asked to eat literally TONS of unhealthy chickens a year.

Stop buying cheap chicken. It's pumped full of drugs and not good for you.

In fact, I would say that eating one of these modern,

fat-breasted, 37-day-old monstrosities is literally gambling with your health.

Buy organic, free-range chicken whenever you can. You'll have better health, and probably better karma in the bargain, too.

MY SIMPLE (AND SAFE) FIX FOR DRY EYE

Modern technology might make life more convenient in a lot of ways, but it sure isn't good for our health.

Case in point: Our excessive exposure to computers, flat-screen monitors, phones, and fake light is terrible for our eyes, and is one of the main reasons why dry eye disease has become one of the most common eye conditions in the U.S.

The symptoms associated with dry eye — dryness, burning, and stinging — can wreak havoc with your quality of life. And if that's not bad enough, over time, it can lead to vision impairment.

I certainly don't blame anyone for reaching for artificial tears. But don't expect them to provide lasting relief because, as with the vast majority of drugs on the market, they don't fix the underlying cause of the problem.

Fortunately, there is a substance found in nature that does get to the root cause of dry eye, and it's something you're already familiar with: omega-3 fatty acids.

One of the main causes of dry eye has to do with poor

tear quality — which omega-3s can help fix.

The tear film has three layers — oil, water, and mucous, and all three need to be present in the right amount to keep your eyes healthy. The oil layer, which is produced by Meibomian glands, is critical because it prevents tears from evaporating too quickly.

Studies have shown that omega-3s increase the amount of fatty acids in the Meibomian gland secretions. Ultimately, this slows the evaporation of the tears, which improves the symptoms of dry eye.

So fish oils, rich in omega-3s, are the answer. But not all fish oil supplements are the same.

A new study has found that a unique form of omega-3s are especially effective in treating dry eye. It's called *re-esterified* omega-3s.

Most fish oils supplements have alcohol added to them to remove toxins from the oil. The problem with this method is that the alcohol converts the fats into a compound that's not easily absorbed by our bodies. When omega-3s are *re-esterified,* it means the alcohol that was added is removed, which makes it easier for the body to absorb.

After 12 weeks of supplementing with this highly-absorbable omega-3, people experienced significant improvements in all of the important measurements associated with dry eye. These include ocular surface disease index, tear concentration, tear break-up time, and omega-3 index levels.

The results were so strong that the researchers recommended omega-3s as primary therapy for dry eye disease.

Finally, a recommendation I can agree with.

AND HERE'S HOW TO STOP GLAUCOMA, TOO...

Glaucoma is the most common eye disease in older people. It is also one of the leading causes of blindness in the world if — and that's a big IF — it's left untreated.

Glaucoma is typically caused by increased pressure in the eye. Over time, the pressure damages the optic nerve, which causes the main symptoms of glaucoma, namely loss of peripheral vision.

The key to combatting glaucoma is to get ahead of it early.

There's just one problem. In its early stages, glaucoma produces no symptoms.

That's why I recommend getting regular eye exams from the time you hit 40 — especially if you're diabetic, have existing eye problems, or have a family history of glaucoma. These are the most common risk factors for glaucoma.

When you get regular eye checkups, your doctor can measure the pressure in your eye. If the pressure starts rising, you can stay ahead of the game by taking steps to lower the pressure before it damages the optic nerve.

In cases where the optic nerve has already become damaged, lowering eye pressure is still key to slowing the progression of glaucoma.

Ultimately, you and your doctor will have to decide if you're going to use prescription eye drops — or even undergo surgery.

But whatever you decide, there are a few natural ways to lower pressure in the eye.

- The first is to get your insulin levels in check. Insulin can increase the pressure in your eye, so one of the best things you can do for your eyesight (and your health) is to cut out the sugary foods, like sodas, sweets, and bread.
- Exercise has also been found to lower eye pressure and improve blood flow to the retina and optic nerve. In fact, these effects can be achieved by raising your pulse as little as 20 percent. These benefits have been seen in both aerobic and resistance exercise.
- One form of exercise I DON'T recommend for people with glaucoma is yoga. While yoga has numerous mental and physical benefits for most people, the inversions that are common in yoga can cause as much as a 2-fold increase in eye pressure.
- Take steps to reduce your stress levels. Just as stress is known to increase blood pressure, it increases eye pressure as well.
- Finally, a handful of nutrients have been shown to protect the optic nerve. These include CoQ10, astaxanthin, bilberry, and magnesium. Also, be sure to eat plenty of seafood for the omega 3s.

BEWARE THIS HUGE SUMMERTIME FRAUD

A few years back I took my wife and three sons on a houseboat vacation on Lake Powell in Arizona.

On any given day you could find us outside the entire day, swimming, tubing, or even hiking through slot canyons.

But I'll tell you what you WOULDN'T find: a single bottle of sunscreen.

That's because, despite convincing ad campaigns by sunscreen manufacturers, there are few things more important for good health than sunlight.

And for the sake of your health, that's important to remember as summer approaches.

Sunlight sets in motion multiple chemical reactions in the body, including activating hormones like melatonin, estrogen, testosterone, adrenaline, cortisol, and insulin, and neurotransmitters like dopamine and serotonin.

And of course, it is hands down the best source of vitamin D. Yet the mainstream has sold the lie that the sun is evil and must be avoided at all costs — and most Americans have bought into it.

The average American spends just 7 percent of their time outdoors — and even then, is covered by clothing, hats, sunglasses — and the worst offender of all, sunscreen.

And we're paying the price.

According to a new article in the *Journal of the American Osteopathic Association,* using sunscreen with an SPF of just 15 or higher reduces the production of the active form of vitamin D (vitamin D3) by a shocking **99 percent.**

These researchers claimed that the combination of sunscreen use plus diseases involving the malabsorption of vitamin D (Crohn's, diabetes, chronic kidney disease) are responsible for causing vitamin D deficiency in more than 1 MILLION people.

Talk about a health disaster.

Low vitamin D levels are one of the biggest risks factors for numerous diseases, including osteoporosis, depression, autoimmune diseases, obesity — and the big ones like heart attacks and cancer.

Vitamin D is necessary for bone health, muscle and nerve function, and the immune system. It is also essential for the proper absorption of calcium, so not getting enough leads to loss of bone density — which naturally increases the risk of bone fractures and osteoporosis.

Instead of avoiding in the sun, we should be basking in it — and that's exactly my advice to you today.

For optimal vitamin D absorption, try to get the sun directly on your skin during the middle of the day. That's when the sun produces UVB frequency, which is the kind that causes the formation of vitamin D.

Keep in mind that the amount of vitamin D provided by the sun will vary by the time of year, your specific location, and numerous other factors.

If you want to know for sure how much vitamin D you're generating, try downloading a free app, like one called

D Minder. It tells you what time of day UVB is present at your location, and it takes into account numerous factors, including cloud cover and skin type.

Just be sure to start slow, especially if you're not used to spending time in the sun. As important as it is to get sunlight every day, it's also important not to burn yourself. It takes about 4–5 weeks of gradually increasing sun exposure for skin to be able to absorb more sunlight without burning.